CULT
STREETWEAR

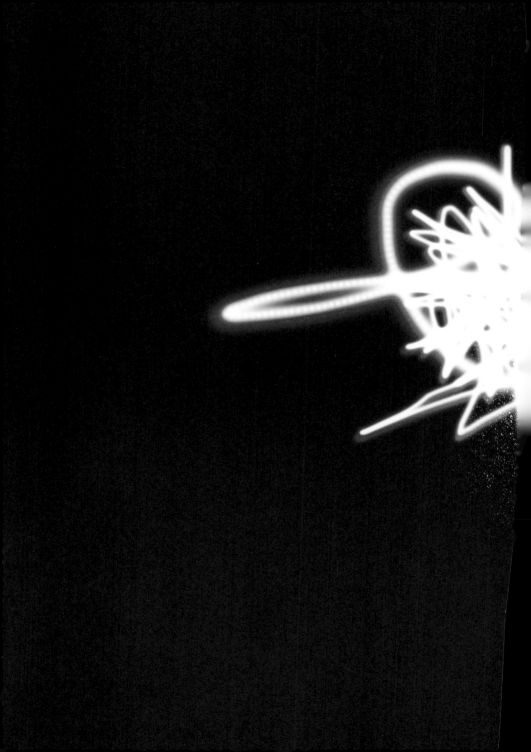

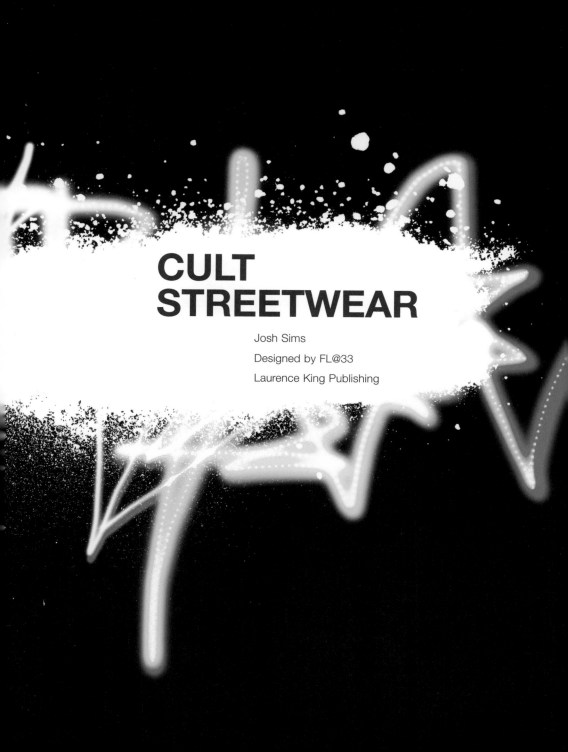

CULT STREETWEAR

Josh Sims

Designed by FL@33

Laurence King Publishing

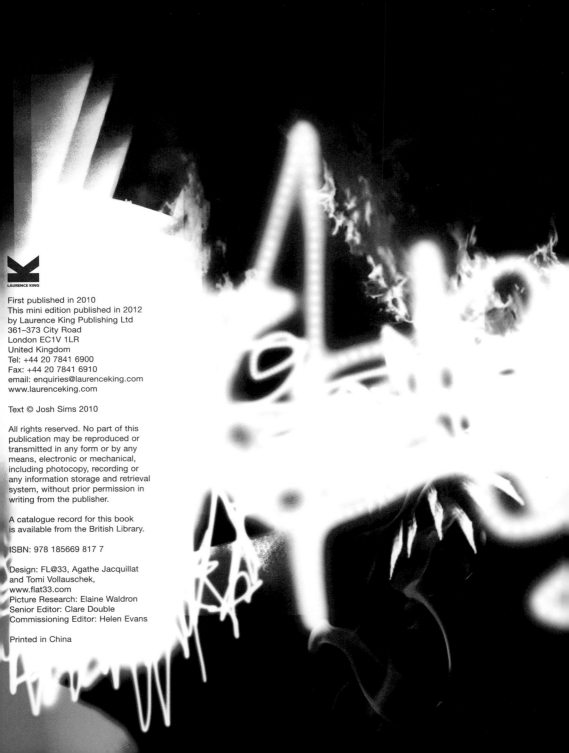

![Laurence King logo] **LAURENCE KING**

First published in 2010
This mini edition published in 2012
by Laurence King Publishing Ltd
361–373 City Road
London EC1V 1LR
United Kingdom
Tel: +44 20 7841 6900
Fax: +44 20 7841 6910
email: enquiries@laurenceking.com
www.laurenceking.com

A catalogue record for this book
is available from the British Library.

ISBN: 978 185669 817 7

Design: FL@33, Agathe Jacquillat
and Tomi Vollauschek,
www.flat33.com
Picture Research: Elaine Waldron
Senior Editor: Clare Double
Commissioning Editor: Helen Evans

Printed in China

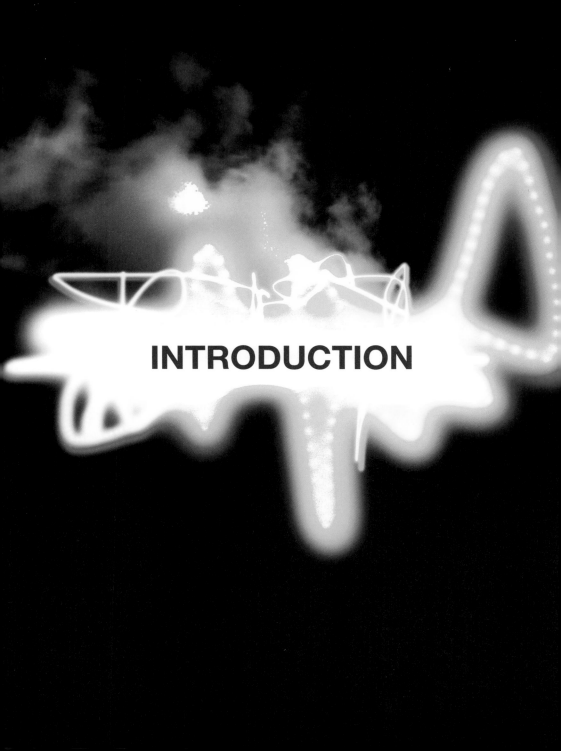

INTRODUCTION

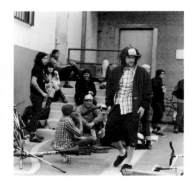

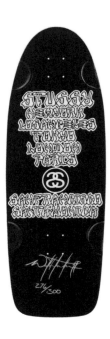

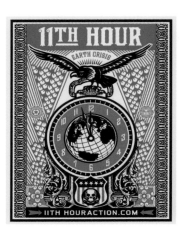

"When people ask what kind of clothes we make, it's always difficult to explain exactly what we do. Usually my answer goes something like, 'Um, we make streetwear'. Which of course doesn't mean much at all. I'm a streetwear company with a certain aesthetic and influences – skateboarding, the LA lifestyle, rap music, rock music. But there's so much more."

When Rick Klotz, the founder of Freshjive, tried to define exactly what his company does and what label to put on it, 'streetwear', rightly, seemed somehow lacking. In part this is because, seen from today's world, in which streetwear has become a catch-all definition for a multi-billion-dollar international market, the word doesn't capture the dynamism of what streetwear both has been and has become; but it is also because streetwear is such a broad church that the very term lacks the precision definition that so many brands require in order to do them justice.

After all, every type of streetwear might share similar inspiration but be interpreted in diverse ways: surfing, skateboarding, BMX, snowboarding – what have come to be packaged as 'extreme sports' – but also the more cerebral pursuits of art and graphic design; punk, with its DIY ethos, but also avant-garde rock, hip-hop and gangsta rap, with its get-rich-quick one; the gung-ho, screw-you hedonism of youth, but also a purposeful, politicized, anti-authoritarian activism; the drive of the African-American working class but also that of the white, art-school-educated and middle class. It has been underground and non-conformist in attitude, overground and over-branded when it comes to making a buck; fuelled by insider knowledge and yet sometimes boastful in its brash oneupmanship; with a foundation in grassroots communities of like-minded people, but often aspiring to corporate power and influence; on the surface as simple, comfortable, functional, practical and much imitated a style of dress as might be imagined, and yet one resplendent with

codes and details that give the apparent clone a strong sense of identity. The t-shirt, the motherlode of all streetwear, is, after all, the ideal blank canvas on which to give vent to one's values, however consumerist they may really be.

This is where streetwear has come from. And so, too, the paths are diverging where it has gone: worn by teenagers, collected by the middle-aged creatives who grew up with it; quintessentially American, and yet co-opted by the Japanese, with the British and Australians, among others, also offering their own take; a story of clothing, but one inseparable from its often obsessive love of imagery, records, gallery-like boutiques and even grown-up toys; a contemporary style of dress that likes to reference the past, that is outward-looking but also self-referential; a home to basic products and yet ones that can command vast sums from die-hard fans; an expression of the environment in which it is created, but also a romanticized, mainstream commodity for those who have no connections whatsoever to that environment; at heart urban and yet everywhere. Streetwear is all these things. And it continues to evolve – now one of the world's biggest fashion markets, it is set to get bigger still, as the product-for-sale is increasingly deemed a viable form of creative expression.

Indeed, as the number of streetwear consumers grows, so does the number of streetwear brands. Every week sees the launch, heralding of and, sometimes, disappearance of the latest arrivals; the media and consumer alike trumpets the latest collaboration or limited edition without much inspection of the (often minimal) creative integrity of the product itself; and the streetwear stereotype – expensive and rare sneakers, baggy denims, hoodie and loose, emblazoned t-shirt – has become an easy uniform for the perma-youthful masses. Once, however, a long time ago in a galaxy not so far away, streetwear was not like

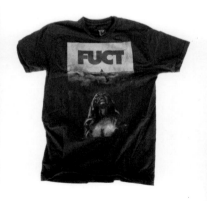

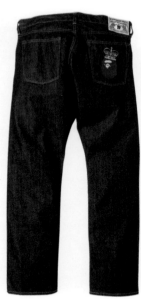

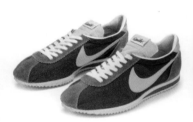

this – it was pioneering. That may be hard to imagine, so ubiquitous is streetwear now. But it broke the fashion mould.

Certainly, if the best of high fashion has been a consequence of the 'trickle up' theory, by which designers interpret the style of the streets for the interests of big business or consumers divorced from its roots; and if the best of street fashion has resulted in movements (each 'streetwear' in its own way), be they punk or Mod, grunge, goth, rocker, skinhead or teddy boy, which defined an era and continue to provide benchmarks and widely understood reference points long after their heyday, then streetwear, as it might be more popularly conceived, has been every inch as influential in the way we dress, if not more so. It has helped to casualize the way we dress, for good.

The difference, perhaps, from prior movements (if such a ragtag and often in-fighting group of different interests can be called this) has been in streetwear's scope. Unlike other movements, which were defined by their exclusivity, it has become a global, inclusive (if inevitably diluted) look, worn by teens, mums, pop stars and paunchy pas alike. Another difference is that streetwear has always been self-determining: if the styles of previous fashion movements have been taken from what was already available, the skill being in the selection of what to appropriate and the way it was reassembled, then streetwear, borrowing from the templates of workwear and sportswear but then running with the idea, built itself from the ground up. In so doing, it became both a major business and a cultish, cultural force in its own right.

From the worlds of industry, sport and that of streetwear itself, *Cult Streetwear* tells the stories of the brands and the people behind them. These are the names that, mostly in the mid-1980s through to the early 1990s (though with some harking back 50 or 100 years), together created the idea of streetwear and to which all subsequent streetwear brands owe a debt. This is true, be they

from mainstream store groups, global, glitzy fashion houses, hip-hop entrepreneurs or increasingly, as these pioneers were, from city back-streets too. The selection of brands in this book is not definitive, as befits a look or an attitude that escapes easy definition. Some choices and some exclusions will, no doubt, puzzle. But, unquestionably, all the brands included here have played a key part in shaping what for some is simply a way to cash in, for others is just something to wear, but for many more is a way of life. Newer brands, a representative few of which are featured, continue to mould streetwear in diverse and surprising ways. They keep the look exciting, just as the pioneers of streetwear did.

Josh Sims

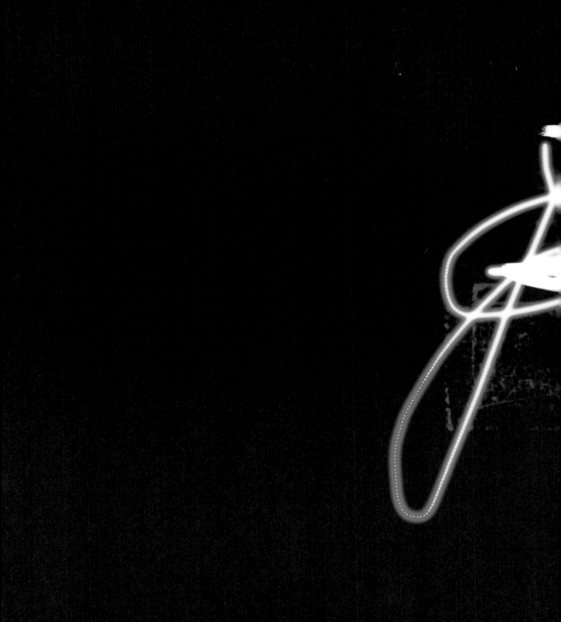

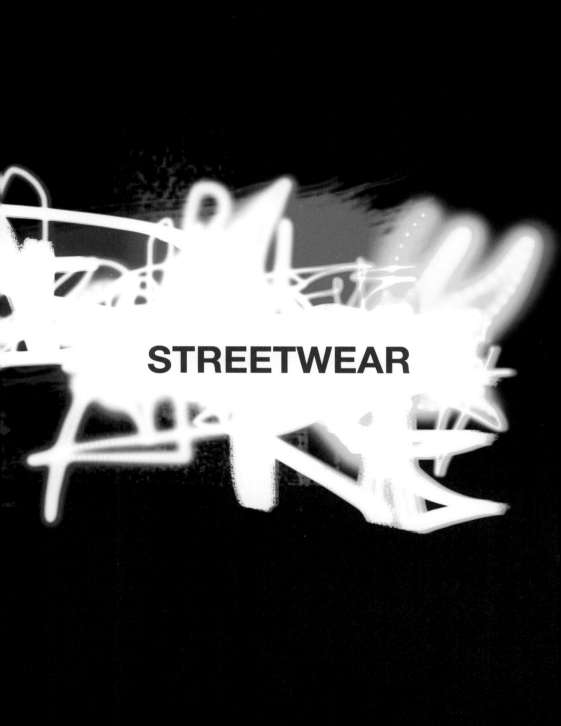

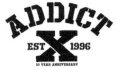

ADDICT®

The port of Southampton, on the south coast of England, may seem an unlikely place to start a streetwear brand. But back in 1994 that was the intention of Addict's founder Chris Carden-Jones, who began with one logo, four t-shirt prints and the aim of creating a British streetwear label – filtered through a more minimalistic, functional sensibility – that could stand up to leading American names in the field.

"Back then I was designing a lot of mixtape covers, flyers and record sleeves," Carden-Jones noted, "and the Addict logo emerged from that time. I'd cut and pasted some text from a magazine spread which included the word 'addiction' for a flyer that I was working on. A few weeks later I cut the word 'addict' from the artwork for a set of t-shirts for a local vinyl store and it was at that point that I first registered the possibility of using the word 'addict' as a brand name to reflect people's loves and passions or positive addictions. We had very little start-up money and no experience of the clothing industry, so we literally started from scratch, using a local printer, buying in the tees and dyeing them to the colours we needed."

Addict grew rapidly from that point, largely through putting on blinkers and avoiding becoming a 'me-too' brand. All patterns, graphics and clothing are still produced in-house, allowing it to follow its own path rather than that of fashion trends. Fabric innovators, including Epic, Japanese denim manufacturers and specialist makers of jackets for the likes of Barbour and Karrimor, have been consulted to ensure that each piece of an Addict collection is as much about substance as style. This association also won the independently designer-owned and -led brand its admirers, and a number of top-flight collaborations followed: with Casio G-Shock (with whom Addict designed camo watches), Vans, Spy Optic snowboard goggles, Canada's Endeavor Snowboard Design, One True Saxon and Sympatex, for technical outerwear.

Addict adds to that a close, long-term working relationship with a number of leading British contributors in the fields of typography and graphic design, among them C-Law, Swifty (designer of the Talkin' Loud and Mo'Wax record label logos), Mr. Jago and SheOne. The result, as the company calls them, are 'Brit hits' (which, like many things British, have helped the brand achieve a cult following in Japan), often packaged as collectibles: including, for example, an artist series of boxed t-shirts featuring illustrations by the likes of Syd Mead, the 'visual futurist' responsible for the looks of films such as *Blade Runner*, *Tron*,

Aliens and *2010*, among other sci-fi movie benchmarks. This was a tie-in that Addict could justifiably call a coup. In common with many streetwear brands, popular culture of the late 1970s and onwards is a particular influence, with Addict producing, among other items, much-imitated *Star Wars* tees.

"The streetwear scene in the UK is still massively influenced by the US, but British streetwear definitely draws its influence from the music and the cultures that we've grown up around through the 1980s and 1990s, such as football casual, the whole birth of sportswear fashion/trainer culture, as well as the huge UK dance music scenes – I think this gives it a different edge and look to its overseas counterparts," Carden-Jones observed. Attention to detail is also, he argued, a British design trait: "The idea behind Addict is to simply produce a good-quality 'real' product that has a high level of design content which doesn't have to immediately jump out at you – it's when you look closer that you see it."

Tie-ins, such as those already mentioned, allowed Addict to set its sights not only on shaping a British answer to US streetwear labels but to compete directly, through expansion into the US market. Compete, but not without respect: the brand's Originator series took the early graphic identities of streetwear brands that informed Addict's launch, such as Freshjive, X-Large and Fuct, and worked them into something new. This was appropriation as celebration. "Already dedicated fans [of such brands], we decided we wanted to do something like that and hatched a plan to create a UK-based clothing company that we hoped one day would sit shoulder to shoulder alongside its US counterparts – the originators who were around from day one and inspired us to do what we do and helped so many other brands to follow," Carden-Jones explained.

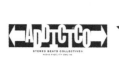
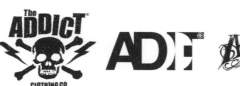
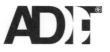

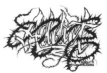
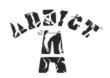

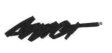

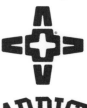

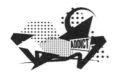

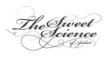
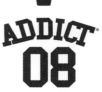

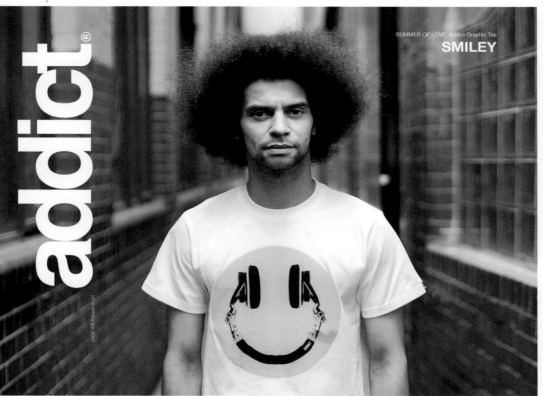

SUMMER OF LOVE. Addict Graphic Tee

SMILEY

The many faces, or rather logos, of Addict (continued over the page). Multiple graphic devices carry the same brand name between collegiate, sporting, rock and roll, tattoo and florid styles.

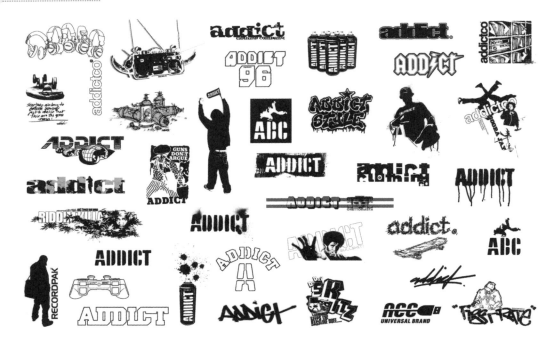

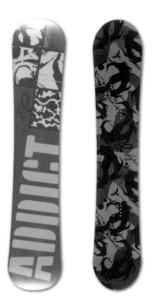
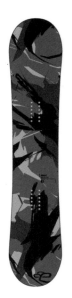
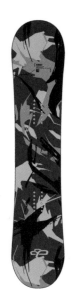
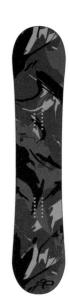
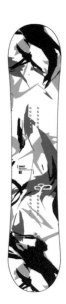

Snowboarding became the natural winter successor to skateboarding. Addict is not alone in seeing snowboards as a repository for its graphic design.

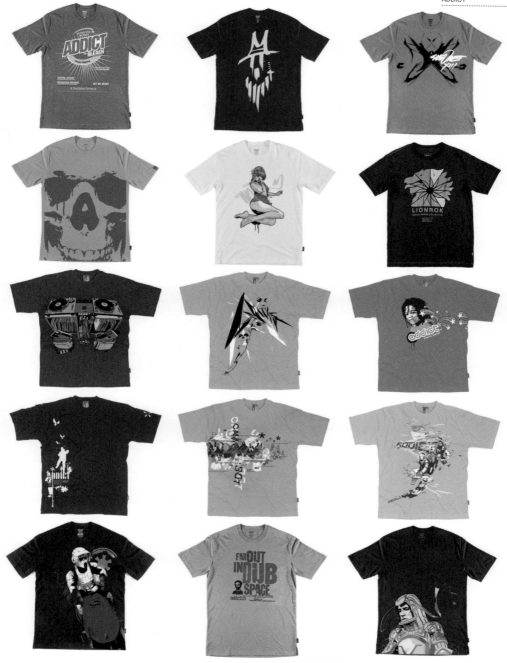

Addict's t-shirt graphics typically make reference to pop culture of the 1970s and 1980s, making them especially nostalgic to thirtysomethings. Here *Star Wars* and *Tron* are among the nods.

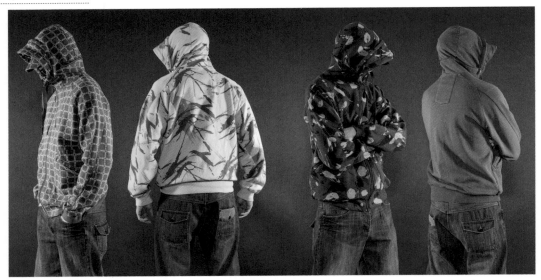

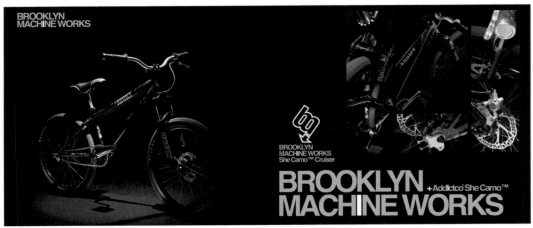

The 'hoodie' has become the definitive streetwear item; lightweight, practical,
midway between sweatshirt and jacket and a site for graphic experimentation.

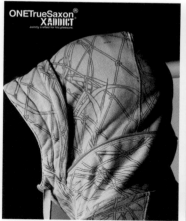

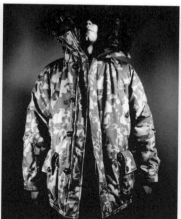

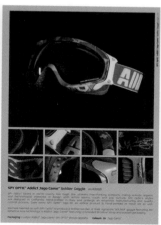

SPY OPTIC® Addict Jago Camo™ Soldier Goggle AU48998

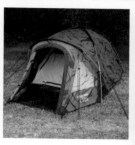

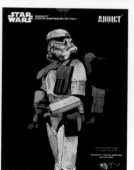

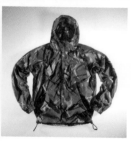

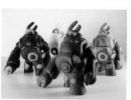

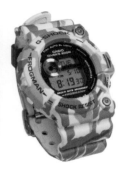

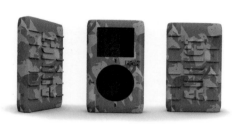

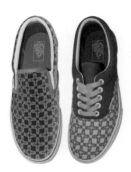

Addict is among the more proactive streetwear brands in collaborating on special products with other brands, among them, here, Casio, Vans, One True Saxon, Spy Optic and, opposite, Brooklyn Machine Works. The Apple iPod case is a prototype that was never manufactured.

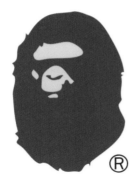

A BATHING APE

Few streetwear brands have ever been in such demand that they need to issue raffle tickets at the doors of their shops in order to select not only who can buy, but what they can buy. But with A Bathing Ape, customers are generally happy to walk away with anything – arguably, A Bathing Ape took over from Stussy as the *ne plus ultra* of streetwear, such that it attracts professional buyers who buy only to sell on at a profit.

But the retail monitoring is in keeping for a brand – better known as BAPE – that has defied convention since it was launched in 1993 by designer-entrepreneur Tomoaki Nagao, aka 'Nigo' due to his similarity to his mentor and Goodenough founder Hiroshi Fujiwara (*nigou* means 'number two' in Japanese). The company has, to date, never advertised or held a sale. Its products are only available through its own stores, complete with sushi-bar-style conveyor belts of sneakers, t-shirt vending machines and other items, notably the signature BAPE camouflage products, which are kept in glass cases like precious *objets trouvés*. Its lines are made in strictly limited editions, with some items available in runs of as few as a dozen, never to be repeated.

This was an approach born of a shortfall of cash when the company was launching. But it grew into a 'keep them keen' philosophy that has more than paid off: the BAPE logo, the head and shoulders stencil of a gorilla, has become the Louis Vuitton of streetwear, and BAPE is the first streetwear brand out of Japan to achieve international credibility akin to that of the country's acclaimed high-fashion designers. Although many different explanations have been given, the brand's logo and name are said to be attributed to a comment made by the designer that Japanese youth had become as comfortable – and in turn as complacent – as an ape bathing in warm water. BAPE came with a DIY-meets-luxury aesthetic to shake the foundations again.

Indeed, it has become a cult brand not only among hip-hop's power base but among creative communities of all ages around the world. It has diversified into womenswear as well as childrenswear, bars, beauty salons, an art gallery, a toy division, a record label – drawing artists including Cornelius and James Lavelle – and its branding exercises have resulted in, for example, every Pepsi can in Japan receiving a BAPE makeover. In addition, there have been collaborations over the years with Nintendo, Disney, Adidas and DC Comics, among others. "It's important for the brand – for fashion brands especially – to be seen to be doing the unexpected. Fashion brands have to stay interesting," as Nigo put it.

Cultishness may be what many brands strive for, but it is not a label that Nigo is comfortable with. "I really fight shy of the idea that A Bathing Ape is like some twisted religion. It suggests that there's something obsessive or sick about it," he said. The fashion writer-turned-designer has sidelines in toy collecting, DJing (even creating a 'supergroup' with a number three hit for the Japanese album chart with "Beef or Chicken") and investing, helping rapper and music producer Pharrell Williams to launch his own clothing line, Billionaire Boys Club.

A Bathing Ape has seen phenomenal growth since Nigo, then a DJ and cool-hunting columnist for a Japanese fashion magazine, first established a small store called Nowhere in Tokyo's Harajuku area with Jun Takahashi, the designer of Undercover. But the store remains very much the product of its frontman's passions: vintage Americana, old-school sneakers, rare vinyl, the kind of precision interests that lead one, in Japan, to be referred to as an *otaku* and to spend inordinate hours searching for very specific fashion treasures. In fact, Nigo remains a manic collector of insatiable appetite, to the extent of seeming eccentric – but the details, colours and heritage often feed back into his collections.

Nigo's first product, as with many streetwear brands, was a graphic t-shirt, with 'Last Orgy II' stencilled around his gorilla proto-logo. The right crowd began sporting, and seeking out, the limited edition t-shirt – of which Nigo sold only five, and gave 25 away – and a market for a counter-cultural label was born. Nigo was a key figure in Tokyo's Urahara scene, which has come to be regarded as a seminal moment in Japan's shifting youth culture akin to the B-boy movement in New York or the Dogtown skaters of Los Angeles. With BAPE, Nigo became the scene's undisputed leader, one of Japan's richest designers and head of the only streetwear brand to emerge from it and achieve an international scope.

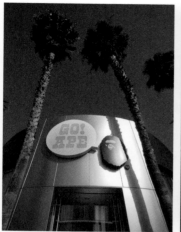
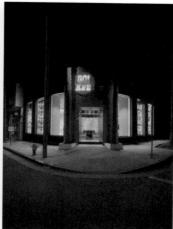
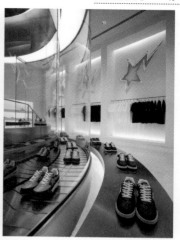

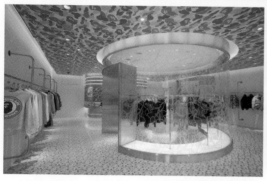
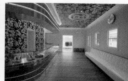
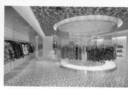
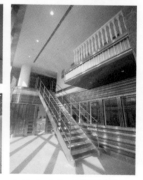

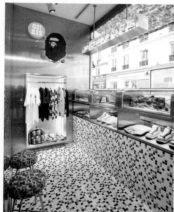
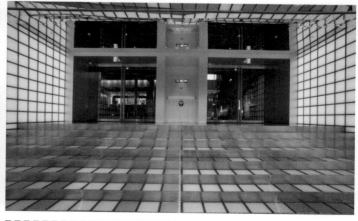

If other streetwear brands aim to keep their store designs as close to the street as possible by using basic materials and an urban decor, A Bathing Ape goes to the other extreme. This is perhaps symptomatic of streetwear's transition from a niche sector appealing to the youth market to a global business selling to grown men (the same youths 20 years on), who perhaps no longer have to wear a suit and tie to work. A Bathing Ape's stores are experiences in their own right, repositioning the clothes as sacred objects.

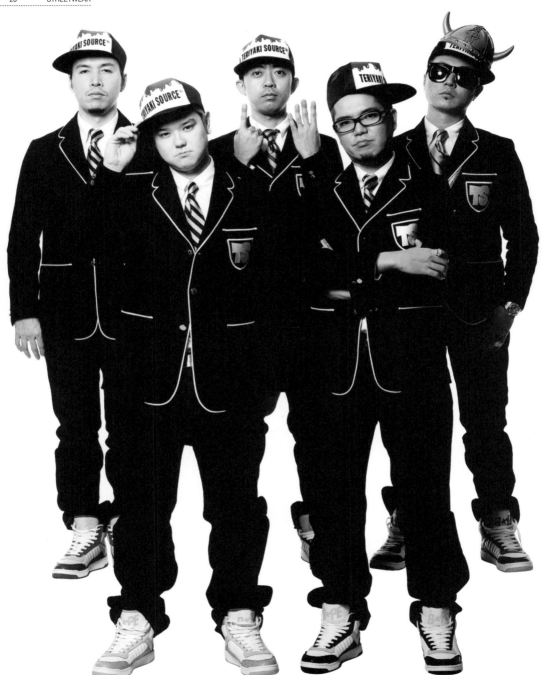

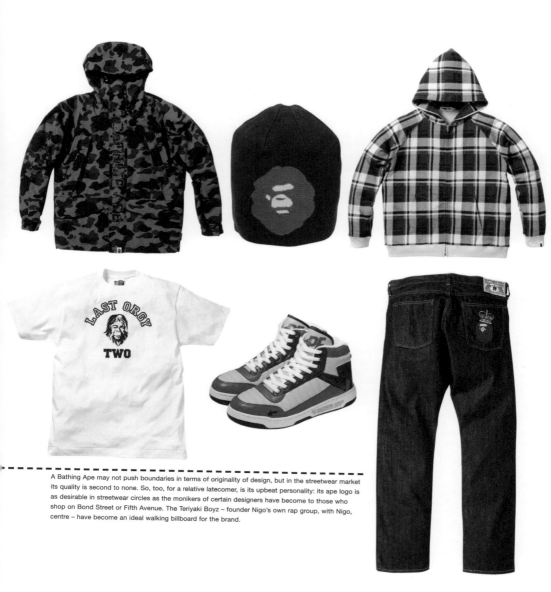

A Bathing Ape may not push boundaries in terms of originality of design, but in the streetwear market its quality is second to none. So, too, for a relative latecomer, is its upbeat personality: its ape logo is as desirable in streetwear circles as the monikers of certain designers have become to those who shop on Bond Street or Fifth Avenue. The Teriyaki Boyz – founder Nigo's own rap group, with Nigo, centre – have become an ideal walking billboard for the brand.

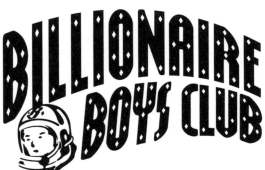

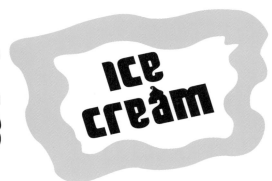

He has won *Esquire* magazine's Best Dressed Man award, been the face of an advertising campaign for Louis Vuitton – leading to a design collaboration on sunglasses and jewellery for the brand – and, as a music producer, has worked with Nelly, Snoop Dogg, Jay-Z, Gwen Stefani, Madonna and Justin Timberlake, not to mention creating music as one half of The Neptunes. Possessing credibility with the streetwear consumer at this level, it was hardly surprising that Pharrell Williams' venture into the street fashion world, with his own lines Billionaire Boys Club and Ice Cream, quickly found success.

In part this is because Williams has a high-pedigree helper: Billionaire Boys Club was co-founded in 2005 by Nigo, the founder of A Bathing Ape, whom Williams met – how else? – through Jacob, jewellery designer to the hip-hop community. The project almost never came to fruition. Williams was due to launch a clothing line in conjunction with sports giant Reebok, but a dispute brought that collaboration to an end in late 2004. Now it would be hard to imagine the two brands without Nigo's handwriting.

Nigo was no doubt drawn to the project because it promised a clothing line with the potential for global wholesale distribution (A Bathing Ape, in contrast, is at the time of writing only distributed through its own stores). But the appeal of Williams' own design aesthetic must have helped seal the deal: a clean-cut preppy style highlighted by candy colours and strong graphics; streetwear crossed with dressier designerwear. Add to this the use of technical fabrics, such as wool and GoreTex blends, together with graphics designed by the underground Japanese street artist (and original BAPE graphics designer) SK8THG, and the package becomes a potent one.

Indeed, Billionaire Boys Club and Ice Cream, it might be argued, are leaders in the field of second-wave, almost post-modern streetwear brands – following the pioneers who built the market but driving it, now it has matured, in new directions that extend its appeal to consumers looking for a more presentable

style and top-flight fabrication. In other words, these are luxury skate lines, including t-shirts, polos, sweatshirts, denim, knitwear, shirts, hats and sneakers, but also underwear and suits. While BBC, as the brand is sometimes abbreviated, is the more slick of the two, Ice Cream (the name was created by combining slang for diamonds, 'ice', and money, 'cream') takes its inspiration more from 1950s Americana (a pet love of Nigo's and one reflected in some Ice Cream store designs, with red-and-white-checked tiling reminiscent of 1950s kitchen interiors or ice-cream parlours). Ice Cream also operates its own pro skate team.

Both lines have ensured some exclusivity by being made in Japan in limited numbers – to order, in fact. That Nigo and, more pertinently, the high-profile Williams often wear the items before they are available to the public only serves to inflate demand. That the clothes are worn by a number of celebrity friends, including Ludacris and Kanye West, fans the flames, with demand further fuelled by stores taking delivery of new stock every two weeks – and fast selling out.

A new brand with more than a touch of retro Americana – as beloved of the Japanese fashion market in particular – BBC and Ice Cream's shop designs jump between nods to space travel (albeit seen through the eyes of a comic book reader) and 1950s ice-cream parlours. Either way, they have a cartoonish intensity to them, much like the clothing.

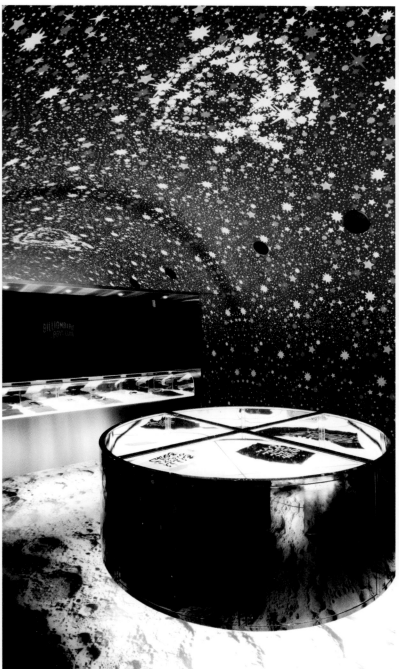

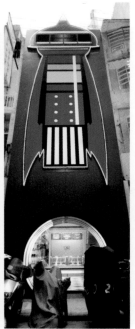

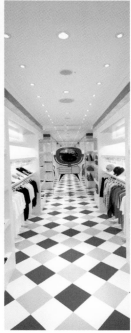

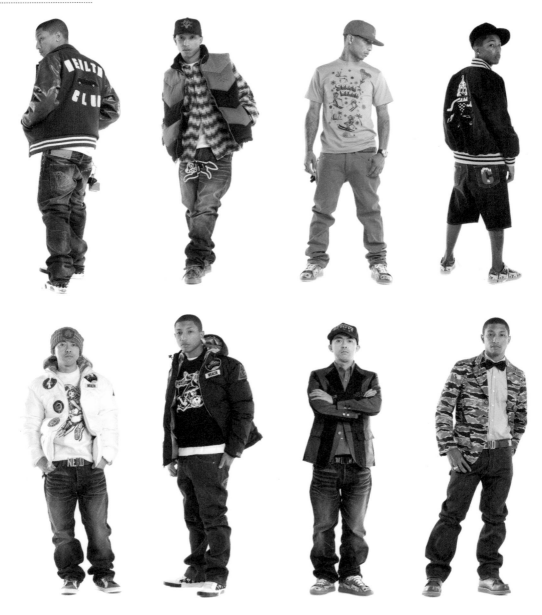

Billionaire Boys Club's designs reference the work of other designers such as Vivienne Westwood, but find their strength in the use of unexpected pattern and graphics. This could be camouflage on a tailored jacket, boating stripes, multiple badges or denim prints with unexpected placing, such as right across the groin (top row second left). Here a number of designs are modelled by the co-designers, Williams and Nigo.

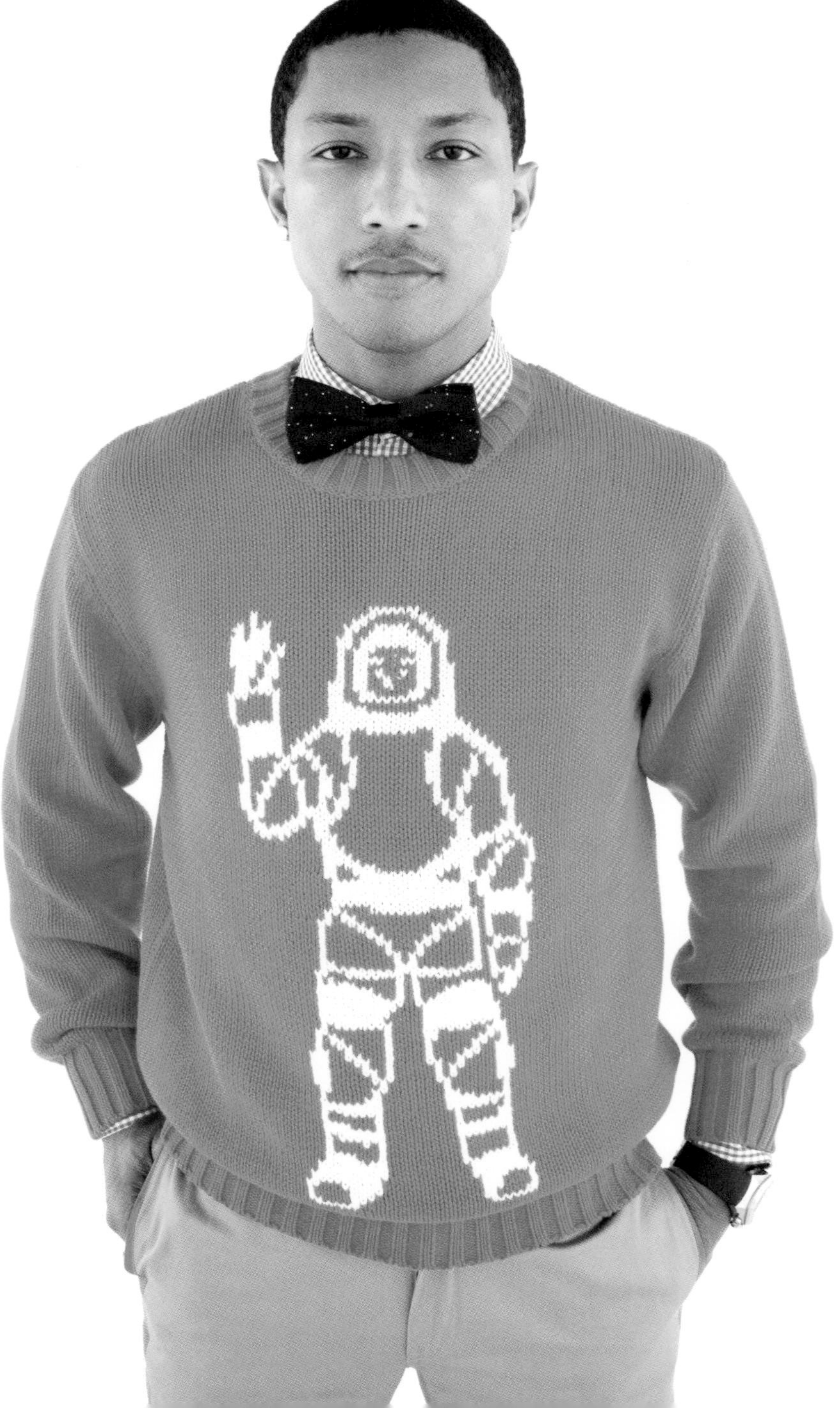

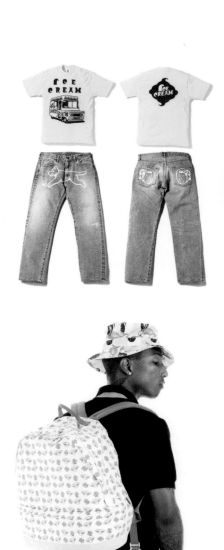

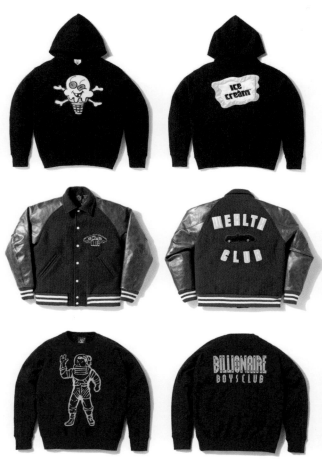

Williams, opposite, in a style more influenced by the quirkiness of Japanese design than the usual East or West Coast interpretation. It's smarter in a preppy way – to the point of parodying smartness.

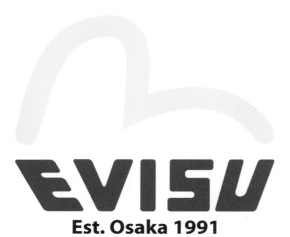

EVISU

Est. Osaka 1991

Denim has been as central to streetwear as the t-shirt or sneakers – blue collar, hard-wearing yet comfortable, improving with age, mass-manufactured and yet individualistic. Ever since Levi Strauss imported *serge de Nîmes* and sewed it up into his five-pocket western style for pan handlers and ranchers of the American West (one Jacob Davis would supply the idea for the rivets), jeans have been the quintessential everyman garment, streetwear demanding them worn loose and low-slung – in homage, it is said, to prisoners in the US who also had to wear them in this way when their belts were confiscated. But, from short-run t-shirt prints to limited edition or deadstock sneakers, streetwear has also sought the one-off and special – and jeans would not escape this kind of attention.

There had long been denim aficionados, of course, who knew their weaves, selvedges and labelling, in the same way as the bon viveur knows fine wines – in Japan they are called *otaku*, people with an obsessive attention to a certain sartorial detail. And so it is fitting that it was in Japan in 1988 that one Hidehiko Yamane, a Japanese tailor by trade, made a few pairs of jeans for his friends. They were hand-finished, made of the best denim available and in the old, post-war style, before mass-manufacturing turned jeans into a commodity product. To ensure authenticity, Yamane even bought the original 1950s shuttle looms from Levi's and insisted that long-abandoned manufacturing techniques, such as indigo loop dyeing and chain-stitching, were reintroduced. Tellingly, the jeans bore the word 'maniac' on their labels.

In 1991 these few pairs of jeans resulted in the launch of a brand, Evis, named after the Buddhist god of prosperity and better known in the West as Evisu (following legal action by Levi's against the too-similar 'Evis' name), and provided a paradigm shift in attitudes to denim. There had been designer denim before. And in Japan there were already other niche denim brands. But with Evisu, suddenly the blue stuff had cachet, credibility and craftsmanship again. Premium denim had been born, and with it (especially among the urban youth of the UK) a new status style – the wearing of a turn-up. This was adopted, not so much to

achieve the right leg-length or to wear prior to shrink-washing as to show off the distinctive selvedge, and a new status logo – Evisu's painted seagull-style 'kamome' insignia across the rear pockets (in homage to the way Levi's painted their back pocket arcuate design, rather than stitching it, during the Second World War to save thread).

"I love the 1940s and 1950s fashion of America," Yamane said. "The fact that the look is still with us shows how strong it was. A special culture for fashion was born around that period: the cloth of the era was of good quality and became the basis of all casual and streetwear, worldwide and not just in Japan."

Evisu's denimhead obsessiveness may seem unremarkable now, but at the time was revolutionary for a staid market. Indeed, it was in large part Evisu's influence that encouraged jeans to be reconsidered not only as a top-end product, but rife for interpretation. It gave artistic licence to more specialist streetwear brands to produce their own lines of typically loose-fitting denims and, as a Japanese brand winning international recognition, helped pave the way for the likes of A Bathing Ape. Although Yamane subsequently expanded his brand in ways that moved it beyond casualwear – even encompassing Savile Row tailoring – Evisu has remained on the periphery of street culture: its golf attire, for example, has been popular with the likes of the Beastie Boys and a new generation of 'punk golfers'.

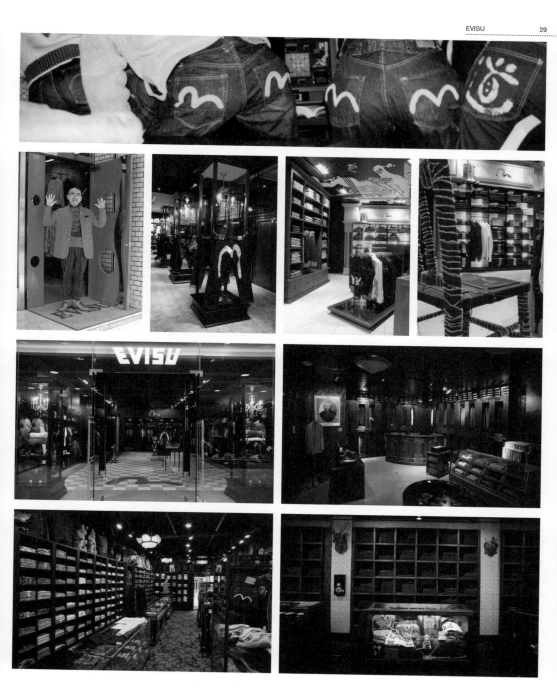

Evisu's store interiors reflect the Japanese love of traditional English style. An old-fashioned haberdasher's feel creates the atmosphere of a gentlemen's club.

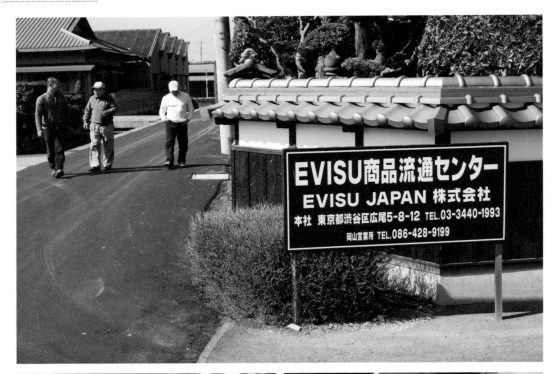

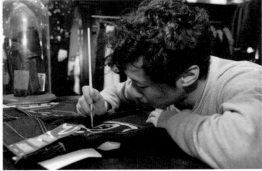

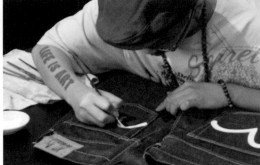

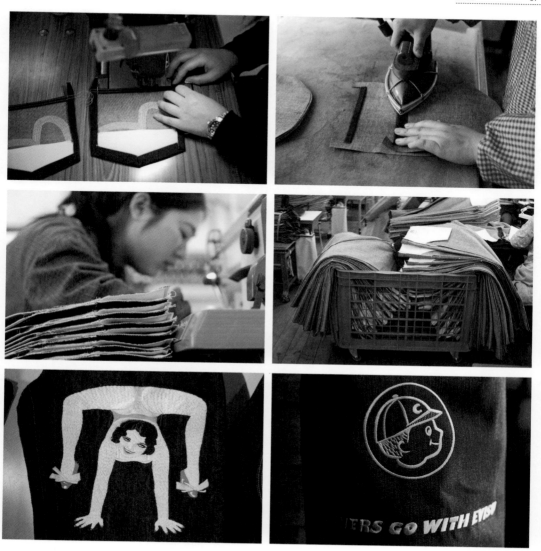

Evisu can lay claim to pioneering premium denim in the early 1990s, and its success has in large part been due to quality standards. The 'arcuate' is hand-painted onto the pockets (opposite), in homage to the methods used by Levi's during the Second World War, when thread had to be conserved for the war effort.

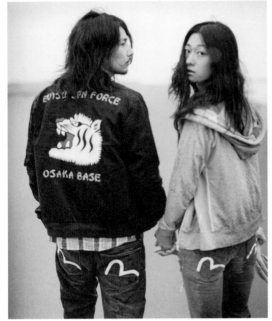
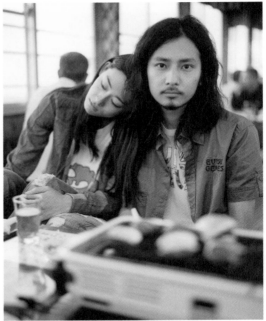
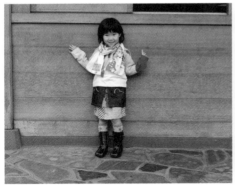
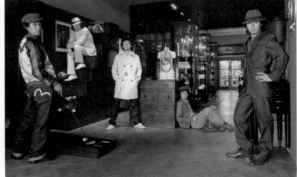
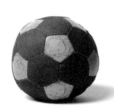
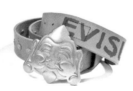
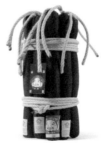
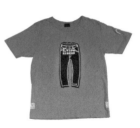

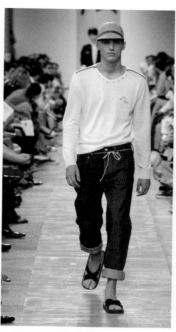
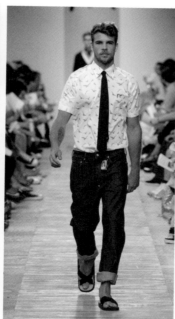
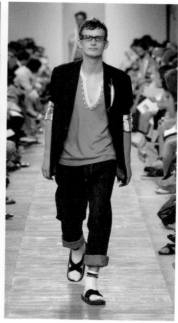

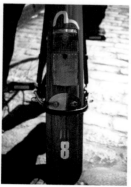
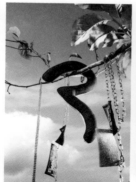
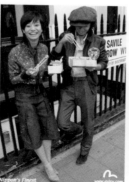
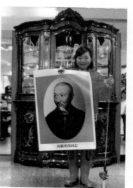

Evisu has extended its streetwear credentials by coming full circle to founder Yamane's early career as a tailor, introducing both catwalk collections, suiting and, symbolically, a store on tailoring's spiritual home, London's Savile Row.

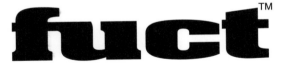

Erik Brunetti likes his designs to be as direct and honest as he is. Few designers, after all, would be willing to produce a Saddam Hussein t-shirt with the caption 'in our hearts forever' that, all irony aside, seems to suggest some empathy with the late Iraqi dictator. "America creates its own super-villains, thus turning them into martyrs – the shirt is clearly depicting that," Brunetti has explained, expressing the kind of political thought that is lost to most fashion. "It's too easy to take pot-shots at dummies. It's like shooting deer in a cage. I enjoy a challenge and a certain amount of brain stimulation."

But it can get personal too, albeit with tongue somewhere in cheek. At one point Fuct, his label, stopped selling to the entire Australian market after extensive troubles with counterfeiting there. "I got fed up with dealing with that type of gypsy mentality," Brunetti said. "I guess I should have expected no less from a country based entirely on a colony of convicted felons." Ironically, perhaps, it is the fact that Fuct designs have been so widely copied over the years that has always pushed the brand to up the ante, using intricate designs and the best available screenprinting methods so the difference between an original item and a bootleg is plain to see.

That has been the case for some years now. Fuct was established in 1990 by graffiti writer and artist Brunetti out of his Venice Beach bedroom, making it one of the few genuine streetwear brands to kick-start what would become a huge market, but also one of the few to capture the renegade sprit of streetwear's early years. These were not just t-shirts for skaters or surfers (though they drew on the visual culture of both, together with that of punk rock) but subversive, counter-cultural statements and, admittedly with some further irony, critical comments on consumer society. Does he feel responsible for the impact of these images and messages? No, he has said bluntly.

Planet of the Apes has been a recurring (and much imitated) motif, but so have references to the Second World War, the Vietnam War and Sioux Indians, not to mention ornithology. And rarely will you find graffiti on a Fuct item. According to Brunetti, graffiti belongs on the street and to commercialize it is to dilute its outlaw message. "It's similar to seeing a once proud, wild panther taken from its natural habitat and put in a zoo – it becomes safe and loses its purpose." He is still a prolific tagger, joking – possibly

– that he pays his taxes and so regards public buildings as fair game. This approach has made Fuct rock and roll enough to win the custom of Keith Richards (no doubt especially pleasing to Brunetti, given that he too is an accomplished guitarist), but sufficiently highbrow to be sported by the artist/film director Julian Schnabel. Indeed, perhaps part of the appeal of Fuct is its high artistic content.

Certainly, on one level the graphics are merely that: graphic, bold, arresting. "I have always admired hunting camo and hunting attire in general," Brunetti has said, by way of example. "The visual of someone wearing Mossy Oak camo fleece [a Fuct design] in the middle of a metropolitan city is uncanny. It's the equivalent of seeing a neon flashing sign in the middle of the forest. I like the dichotomy." But on another level they push at the edges where Brunetti's more personal, non-commercial art begins, in which, it seems, he finds much greater fulfilment and for which he has, it also seems, much greater respect. He has dismissed much of what has been offered by way of streetwear graphics during the intervening years since Fuct launched as 'novelty', more an expression of what the latest computer design technology makes possible rather than of personal insight or conviction.

"Twenty years from now, it will not hold any sort of social value in any context whatsoever. It's not pure. It's all ego-driven," Brunetti has said of it, laying down a challenge to graphics-driven streetwear brands. And, he added, "Fuct is merely applying graphics to t-shirts, which, for me, comes easily. The only requirement is having good taste and if you have that you are already light years ahead in this industry." Fuct is, of course, more than mere good taste. That is what has kept it more the leader than the follower.

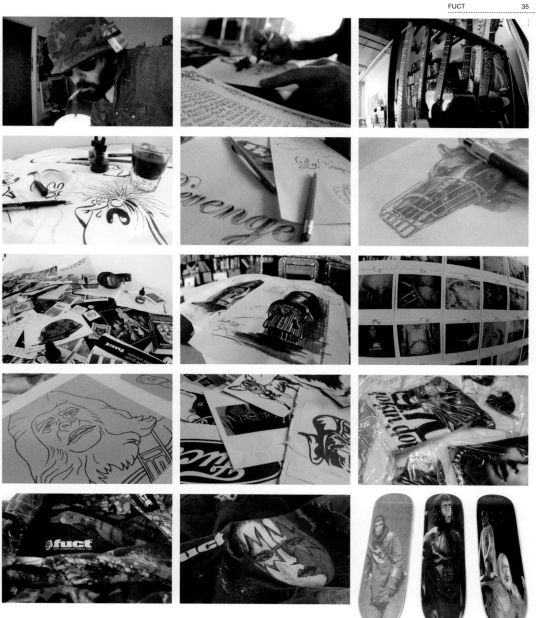

Erik Brunetti in combative spirit, together with the inked-up sketches ready for development as t-shirt graphics. The glam-rock band Kiss and film *Planet of the Apes* (1968) are frequent references – with images from the movie transferred direct to snowboard designs.

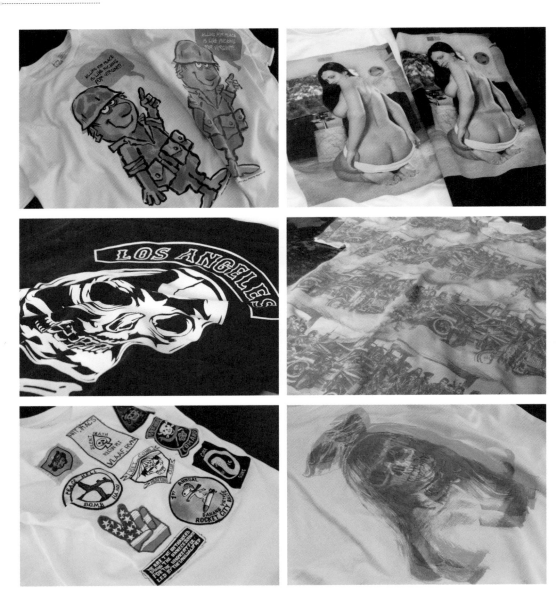

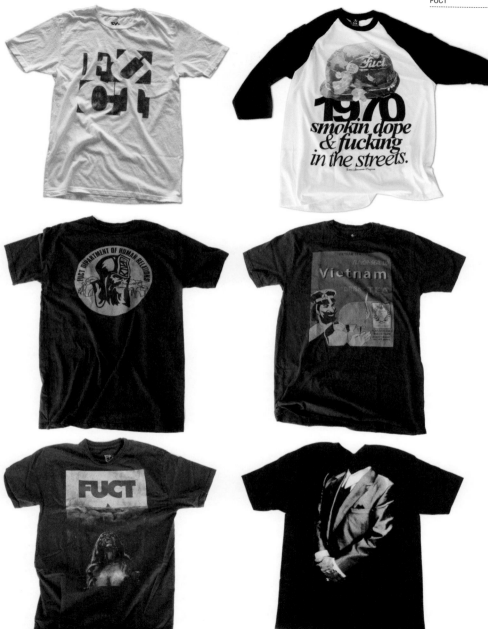

With references from Vietnam to porn, *Jaws* to *Goodfellas*, Fuct's graphic designs run the gamut of pop culture, but typically have some element of socio-political commentary too, from the explicit to the more subtle: 'Fuct Department of Human Relations' reads as much as a dig at society's fallibility as it does a nod to a much-loved sci-fi film.

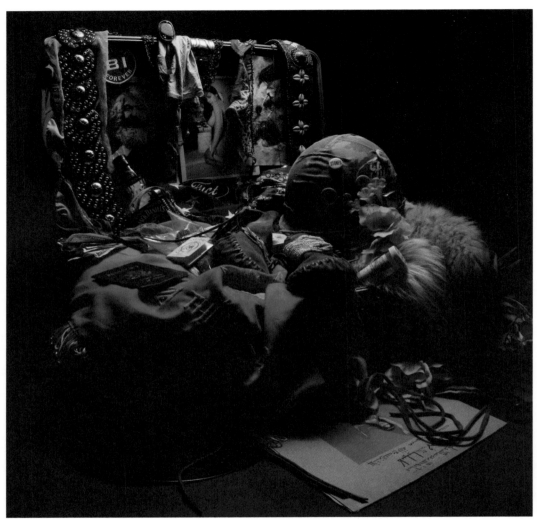

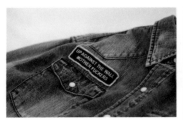

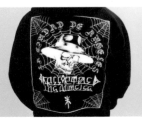

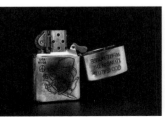

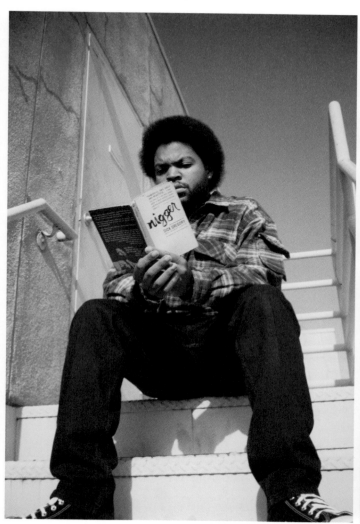

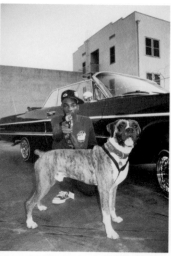

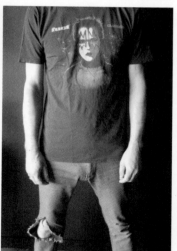

Fuct's love of the iconography of the 1960s and 1970s has led to collaborations with the likes of Zippo, opposite. 'God is alive, living in the White House', reads the inscription. As well as being a leader in graphic design for t-shirts, Fuct has also commissioned photographers to take arresting images for printing onto them. Shawn Mortensen's shots of rappers and streetwear aficionados Ice Cube (above left) and Snoop Dogg (top right) were added to t-shirts for one collection.

GOODENOUGH

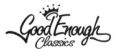

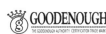

He has been described as a mix of Karl Lagerfeld and Peter Pan and his celebrity in his native Japan is such that his likeness has been recreated as a collectible vinyl toy. But, whichever way you cut it, Hiroshi Fujiwara, and his company Fragment Design, is an undisputed leader of Japanese streetwear, rivalled only for import by Hysteric Glamour's Nobuhiko Kitamura. Here, after all, is the man behind the eclectic accessories brand Head Porter, which became symbolic of stealth chic. He is also the founder of the Electric Cottage label and streetwear brand Goodenough, launched in 1988 and which, although Fujiwara ceased his involvement a decade later, was instrumental in encouraging the streetwear market to address the needs of post-skate grown-ups. Meanwhile, his web magazine, Honeyee, has become one of the most heavily hit street and pop-culture zines and, since 2001, his Base Station retail operation has provided Japan with detailed basics.

On top of this Fujiwara has also gone beyond channelling Harajuku style to become a world-class tastemaker, whose opinion is deemed definitive by international brands and who, arguably, pioneered the now rife ideas both of limited editions (a clichéd idea, he has since claimed – "People are getting tired of collecting things") and streetwear brands working in collaboration. Among his carefully vetted collaborations have been those with Comme des Garçons, Neighborhood and Jun Takahashi's label Undercover, plus big guns Burton (leading to the iDiom label), Levi's (Fenom) and Nike (HTM).

"When I finished Goodenough I realized that I didn't really want to have my own team, whom I have to take care of. So I decided that my company would be me and my assistant, the two of us maybe working with partners, and this is the strategy I'm working with – getting percentages from the projects with the big companies," he explained. "Maybe if I did it myself I could make more money. But I don't want to take the risk. I always wanted to shrink the work a little bit. But that never worked. I don't think anyone knows 100 per cent what I do. I don't even know. But I kind of like it this way."

While establishing his status as collaboration king Fujiwara mentored Nigo, of A Bathing Ape, made music with Eric Clapton (as well as created the artwork for the DVD), and played a cameo role in Sofia Coppola's debut film Lost in Translation. By all accounts he could be very big – as big, for example, as A Bathing Ape – and yet has chosen to stay independent and underground, albeit in a position of extreme influence. "I don't really want to be that famous," he said. "I just want to be kind of mysterious."

His pursuit of the new is driven, in part, by a low boredom threshold: "I always get depressed if something gets really popular. I want to stop, but on the other hand you can make money, so what should you do? I'm always faced with this decision. And I always stop." But it is also a reflection of his interest in being diverse – he is not only a bike fanatic, punk historian, DJ (driving the early popularity of hip-hop in Tokyo) and designer but also a successful music producer and musician. He turns these interests into commercial opportunities, he said, because he does not wait for the market to tell him that they are 'cool'. They simply appeal to him and that is enough. "I only care about now."

"Success [in these fields] is kind of easy because I'm only interested in the things that I like," he has said of his role as street-culture soothsayer. "You know some people may think 'Oh wow, I like the same thing as him', but I liked it already six months ago. They wait until someone pushes it but they hesitate to express their like of something or some brand until maybe I say something about it. I just find something I like and I try to show it. I'm no businessman. The Japanese are good at picking up interesting things and tweaking them to create their own originals," he explained, with some understatement.

Goodenough's simple G logo has the benefit of being easily transferable to a badge or pocket detail, but sometimes the full brand name breaks out. It is testament to the brand's collectible nature that what are essentially classic checked shirts are enhanced by their being emblazoned with the Goodenough name in a way characteristic of fashion in the 1980s.

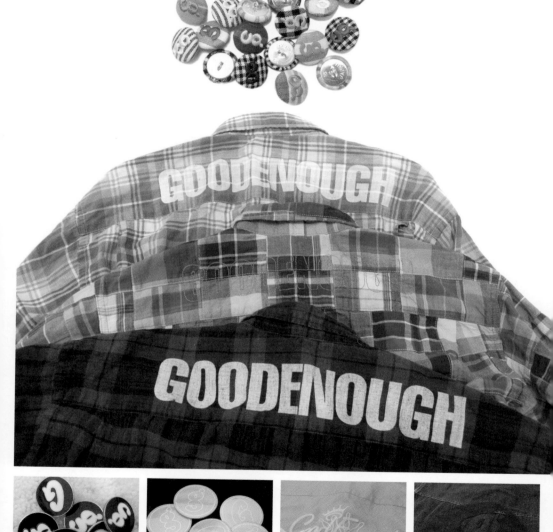

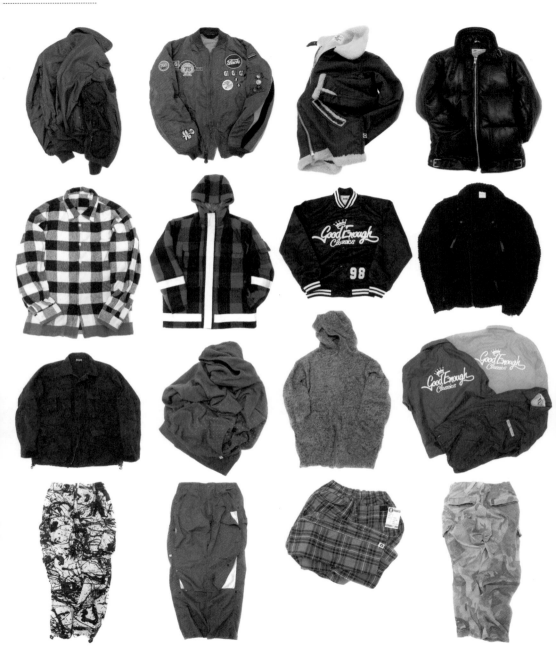

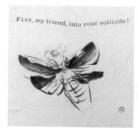

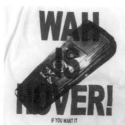

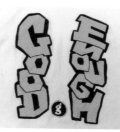

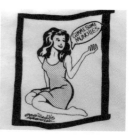

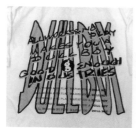

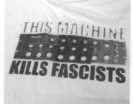

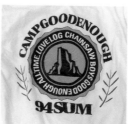

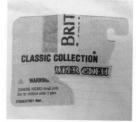

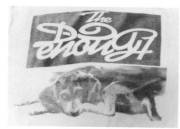

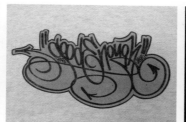

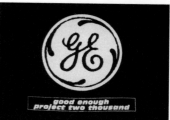

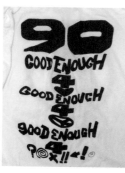

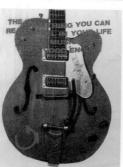

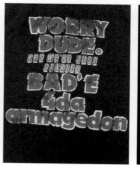

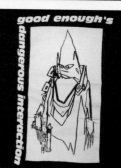

Goodenough, like many streetwear labels, produces t-shirt graphics based on the theme of its own brand name, as here, with the reworking of the General Electric logo (third row right). But the brand's strength lies in its contemporary updating of menswear classics in high-quality materials, such as the combat trousers and baseball, puffa and MA-1 jackets opposite.

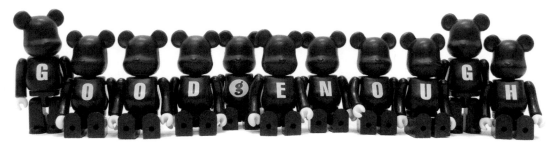

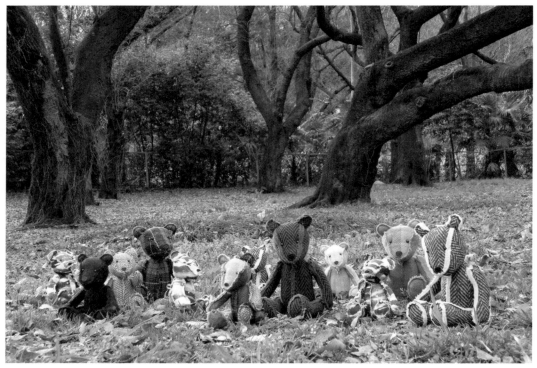

Goodenough has long extended its range beyond clothing, encompassing special projects such as the electric guitar (opposite top) and collaborations with Casio and Japanese bag manufacturer Porter. It has also entered the toy market – not toys for children, of course, but for adult collectors with a latent adolescent streak.

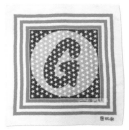

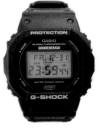

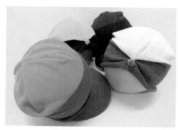

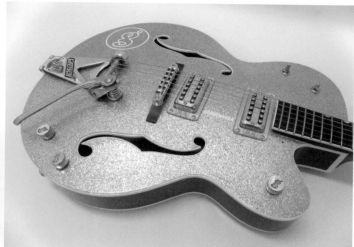

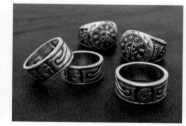

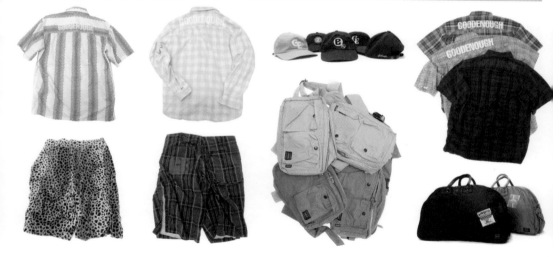

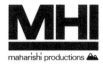

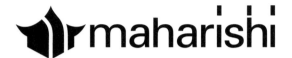

DPM
MHI
DPMHI

It must be, by turns, rewarding and frustrating to see one of your designs copied by almost every fashion retailer on the high street. This fate befell Hardy Blechman, the founder and owner of Maharishi, one of the most influential streetwear brands to originate in the UK. Blechman's roots were in trading recycled workwear and military surplus (both backbones of streetwear), together with the production of hemp/natural-fibre clothing, prefiguring streetwear's growing interest in ecological concerns.

His trading was hand-to-mouth: container shipments of surplus clothing that, due to red tape, had to be sold off asap or scrapped, with Blechman receiving 50 per cent of any sale he could make. There was certainly no shortage of surplus. As he noted, countries with national service, such as Italy and Israel, have to provide new uniforms on a regular basis to what, in effect, are temporary members of the military: once service was completed, the individual's uniform – though usually still in very good working order – is typically declared unusable, it being considered psychologically disadvantageous to pass on a used uniform to a new recruit. Secondly, there has been the military's need to constantly update their uniforms, making 'old' ones defunct. Developments in technology or changes in equipment often necessitate a uniform revamp – and it is undoubtedly the up-to-date functionality of much military clothing that has proved inspirational to streetwear designers.

The experience gave Blechman both a business nous and an appreciation of functional design, while a spell working for a high-street company gave him a distaste for unoriginal design. Little wonder that he considered launching his own line. He did so in 1995 with the military-style Snopant. These were based on military over-trousers used in Arctic conditions, and had a loose-fitting, toggle-adjustable waist, with side button fastenings to allow the legs to be drawn up to three-quarter length (ideal for skateboarding) and were typically decorated with intricate embroidery. It was a midway point between combats and jeans. As well as becoming Maharishi's signature and a global celebrity staple – it was a trademark look for girl bands of the early 1990s – it also 'inspired' endless unauthorized versions.

Many legal wrangles followed. But Blechman's best answer was to give full vent to his obsessions – among them orientalism, camouflage and collecting – and expand the brand into a full collection in 1999, winning him the British Fashion Council's

'Streetwear Designer of the Year' award the following year. Camouflage, indeed, has always been big with Maharishi, and although other designers utilized it in a fashion context before – Stephen Sprouse, Jean-Charles de Castelbajac, Franco Moschino and Richard James among them – few have been quite so militant in their desire to reappropriate it from its military associations.

"I believe that we can guide and change the symbolic meaning of objects," Blechman said. "When you see camouflage now, you think of war. But although the military didn't recognize it, human beings have an instinctive attraction to camouflage – a yearning for unity with nature." For Blechman, camouflage has its roots in bark patterns and animal prints before it does the armed forces. This explains why the military origins of many of Maharishi's pieces are so often subverted by being overlaid with images of eastern mysticism, from 'om' signs to bonsai trees. It is what Blechman has also referred to as "a piss take" – but then his clothes, made at a dedicated factory in Delhi, India, are also smudged with incense, washed in saffron and chanted over in order to help purify any militaristic leanings.

To cement his growing reputation in the market, Blechman later launched mhi, a second line of exclusive designs, incorporating the work of established graffiti artists such as Kaws, Futura 2000, Rostarr and Sharp. He also opened a flagship store in London that became a destination as much for fans of rare Japanese toys and action figures as clothing.

Hardy Blechman, Maharishi's founder and expert in camouflage – as employed by the armed forces, nature and in fashion. All types of camouflage are celebrated in his definitive book on the subject, *DPM (Disruptive Pattern Material)*, seen overleaf, including his own camouflage designs for clothing and store interiors.

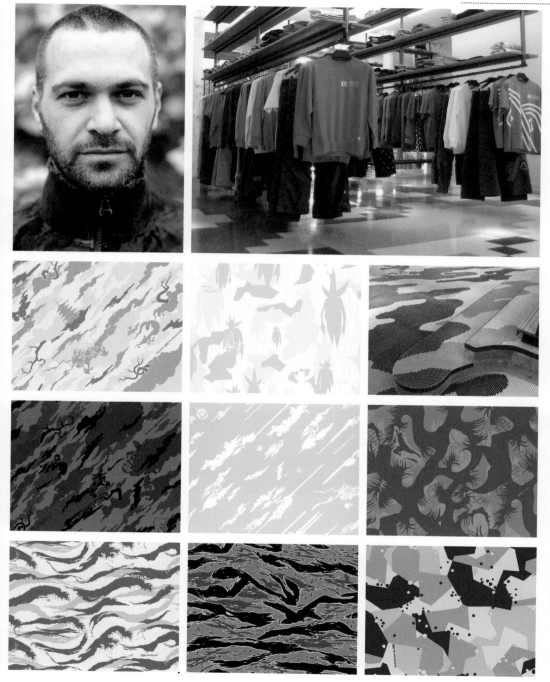

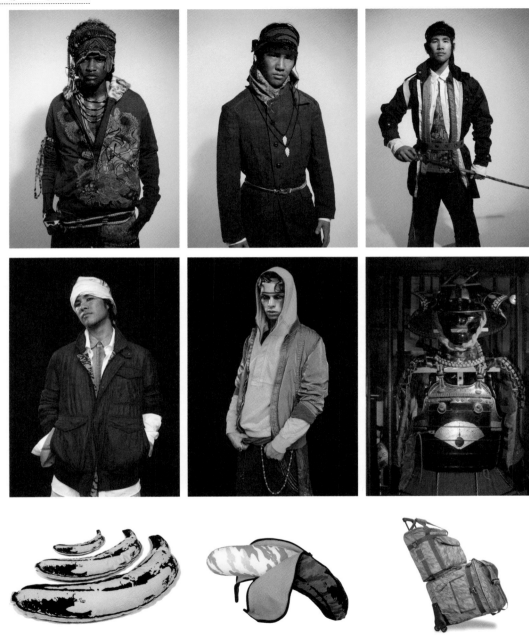

Styles from the Maharishi archive, in part inspired by traditional Japanese samurai dress. Andy Warhol too has proven a frequent touchstone for the brand. The camouflage banana soft toy here was taken from the screenprint the artist made for the cover of "The Velvet Underground & Nico", the band's debut album (1967). See also the Warhol figures overleaf.

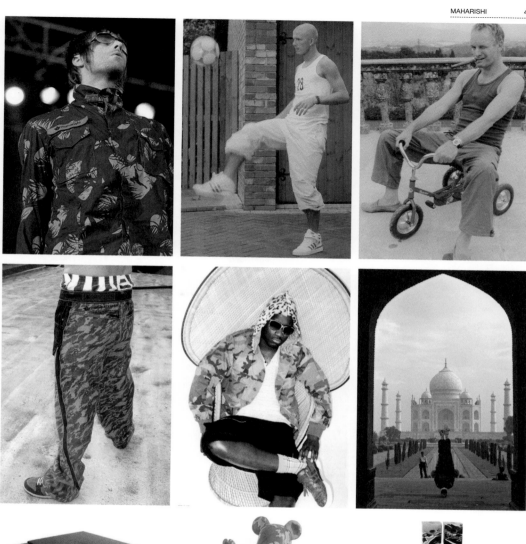

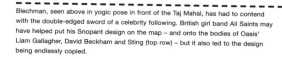

Blechman, seen above in yogic pose in front of the Taj Mahal, has had to contend with the double-edged sword of a celebrity following. British girl band All Saints may have helped put his Snopant design on the map – and onto the bodies of Oasis' Liam Gallagher, David Beckham and Sting (top row) – but it also led to the design being endlessly copied.

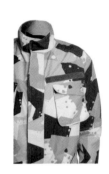

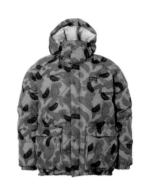

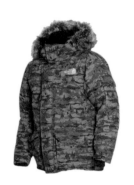

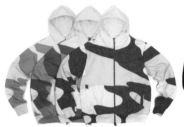

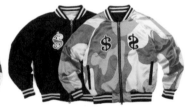

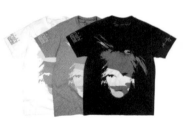

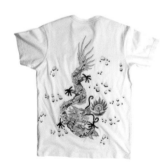

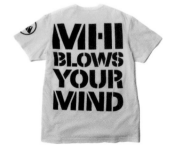

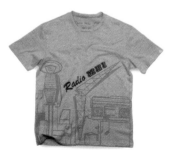

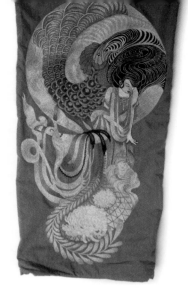

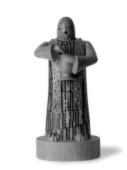

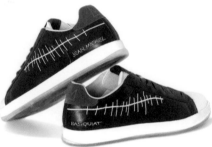

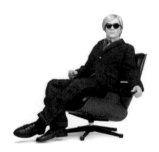

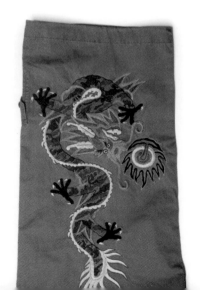

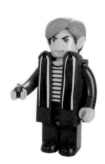

A signature style for Maharishi is the often intensely detailed embroidery found in some versions of the Snopant, shown here with Art Nouveau and Chinese dragon designs. Again this look is widely imitated, albeit with much poorer quality.

MAMBO®

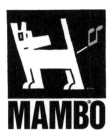

When Mambo was launched in 1984 by businessman and surfer Dare Jennings its intention was quietly subversive: to undercut what Jennings saw as a tendency by the surf market to take itself too seriously. Through a combination of irreverent humour and social and political awareness, Mambo became one of the first brands to transcend its original market and become as recognized in streetwear as it was in surfwear.

In part, Mambo – an abbreviation of a Latin phrase found on the back of a medal presented to Elvis Presley by the US President Richard Nixon – was able to grow through the early support of Phantom Textile Printers, a screenprinting business also owned by Jennings. This backing allowed Mambo the financial freedom to operate on its own terms, often in defiance of market trends. This did not stop it being recognized as a brand of authenticity in its home market of Australia.

Throughout its history, Mambo's humour has been as sophisticated as it has been, as Jennings once put it, "of the toilet kind". In 1990, musician and visual artist Reg Mombassa created Australian Jesus, a 'common-man deity' who reflected the community's general ambivalence to organized religion while at the same time recognizing the influence of Jesus as a historic figure. 'Aussie Jesus' inevitably became a divisive character, as loved as he was hated.

At the less witty end of the graphic spectrum is Mambo's iconic Farting Dog. Nearly 20 years after first appearing on a Mambo t-shirt – and shortly before being temporarily retired in 2005 in a bid by Mambo to pursue a trendier image – the dog, the company noted with characteristic off-beat humour, had earned more than the annual GDP of the former Russian state of Azerbaijan.

A reputation for kicking society's sacred cows has never prevented Mambo from being considered seriously, however. In 1993 Mambo was invited by the Australian National Gallery to exhibit beside an international collection of Surrealist art. Similar shows followed, both at home and abroad. Along with original art by regular contributors such as Richard Allan, Maria Kozic, Paul Worstead, Matthew Martin, Mark Falls (US), Rockin' Jelly Bean (Japan) and Steve Bliss (UK), exhibitions featured company-designed CD covers, books, surfboards, posters and ceramics. These shows often attracted record crowds, drawn by an aesthetic perhaps epitomized by the Mambo Loud Shirt, the company's take on the classic Hawaiian shirt.

Similarly, in 2000, a year before Jennings was to sell his company to a Sydney-based clothing manufacturer, Gazal Industries, Mambo was invited to design the Australian athletes' uniforms for the opening ceremony of the Sydney Olympic Games. While the uniforms themselves attracted wide praise, the decision to become involved in such a mainstream event upset many of Mambo's core supporters. Jennings would later call it his "poisoned chalice".

Indeed, Mambo consistently undercut its move from small-scale streetwear label to lifestyle brand, perhaps uncomfortable with the pomposity that such a definition might imply. 'More a pair of shorts than a way of life' was the byline for one early ad. On another occasion Mambo controversially used a childrenswear swing-tag to encourage parents to 'Buy your children's love with a gift from Mambo'. More controversial still was a poster by Richard Allan featuring a young bike rider laying splattered beneath the wheels of a truck. Above the vehicle appeared the words 'Live fast die young in a nice pair of shorts'. While the poster drew howls of outrage from the California Department of Transportation, an Australian state government used it in a campaign to encourage kids to wear cycle helmets. "Some of our satirical humour has tended to go over the heads of American consumers, who seem happier being fed a diet of Nike hyperbole," noted Jennings.

After being acquired by Gazal, Mambo underwent a makeover in a bid to restore the credibility of a brand which, still being worn by its original fans, had come to be regarded as middle-aged, its once outrageous imagery more passé than provocative. While this makeover attracted the attention of a newer, younger group of fans, it also alienated many of Mambo's original supporters. In 2008 the brand was again sold, this time to an independent group of surf- and street-savvy entrepreneurs, who took Mambo forward by adding to the list of original graphic design stars a new generation of young and talented artists and designers.

"All of my enthusiasm was thrown into Mambo. When it first started, I loved surfing, I loved art, and I had an independent record label so music was something I was close to and (when it came to these things) I knew what I was talking about," said Jennings. "It wasn't a fashion I was pursuing. I came out of the 1970s and the whole Vietnam era so everyone I knew was inherently political. Mambo quickly became an outlet for my various passions."

Part kids' cartoon, part zany funfest, Mambo's style has a surrealist quality that, while off-beat, sometimes verges on the disturbing (or disturbed). Like many streetwear graphics, some of Mambo's co-opt and twist established signage, such as these (bottom row) for hazardous waste warning and washing powder. Others, such as the swing-tag, ironically undercut consumerism: 'Buy your children's love with a gift from Mambo.'

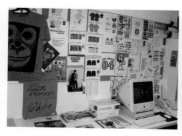
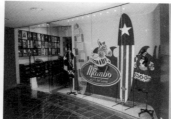
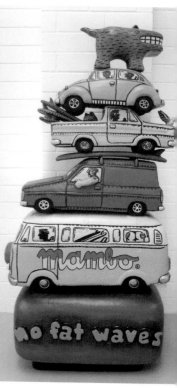
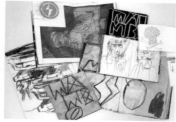
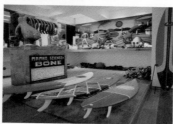
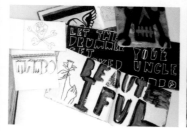
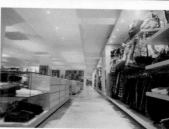

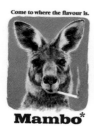

Come to where the flavour is.

Mambo*

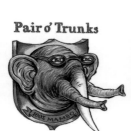

Pair o' Trunks

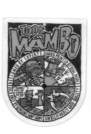

100% MAMBO

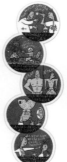

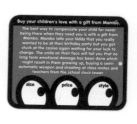

Buy your children's love with a gift from Mambo.

The best way to compensate your child for never being there when they need you is with a gift from Mambo. Mambo tells your kiddy that you really wanted to be at their birthday party but you got stuck at the casino again waiting for your luck to change. The smile on their face will tell you that no long term emotional damage has been done which might result in them growing up, buying a semi-automatic weapon and shooting at class mates and teachers from the school clock tower.

size   price   style

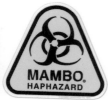

MAMBO.
HAPHAZARD

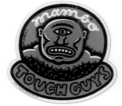

mambo
TOUGH GUYS

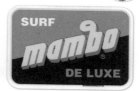

SURF
mambo
DE LUXE

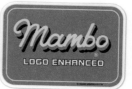

Mambo
LOGO ENHANCED

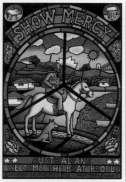 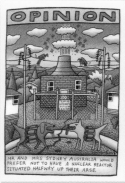 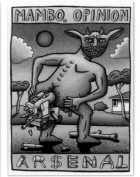 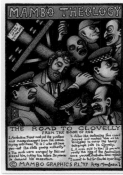

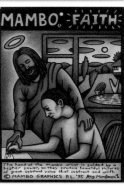 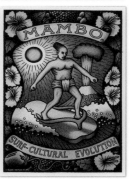 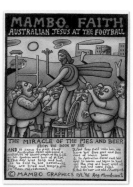 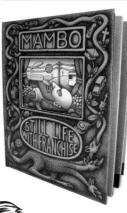

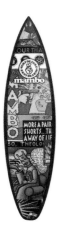 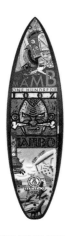 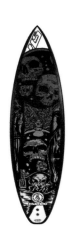 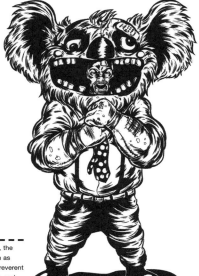

With work by David McKay, Trevor Jackson and Robert Moore, among others, the graphic art of Mambo is in demand for museum and apartment walls as much as fashionable chests. It is hardly surprising that much of its content has been irreverent and combative, raising questions over nuclear power, immigration, armaments and religion. 'Forgive them father', asks a Christ mouse on the cross, 'they know not what to wear.'

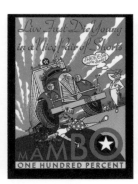

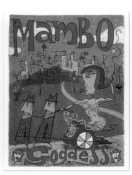

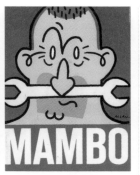

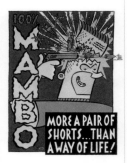

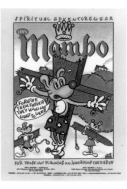

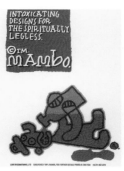

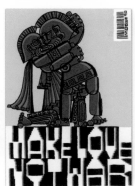

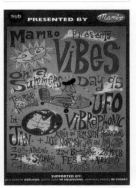

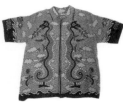

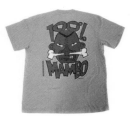

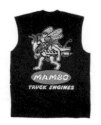

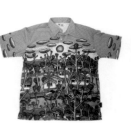

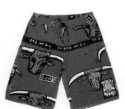

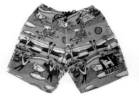

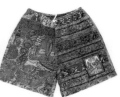

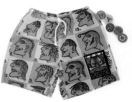

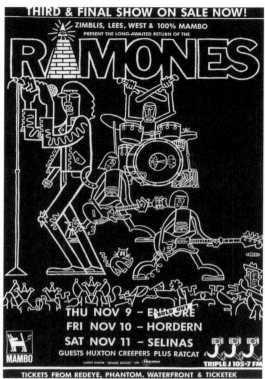

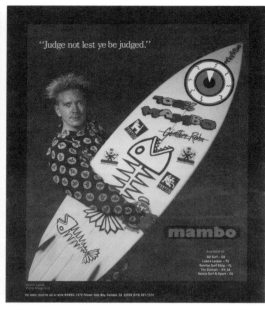

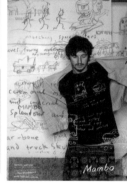

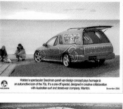

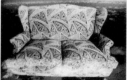

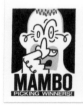

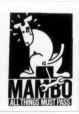

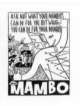

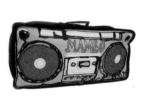

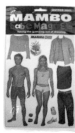

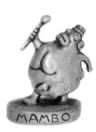

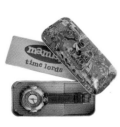

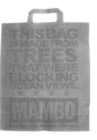

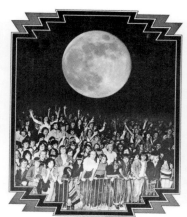

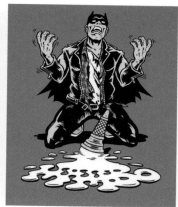

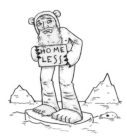

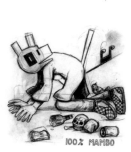

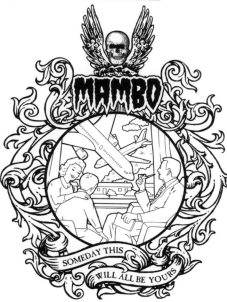

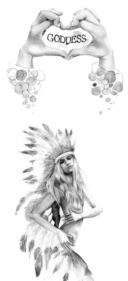

Mambo hiring John Lydon, aka Johnny Rotten of the Sex Pistols, may have been one controversial character meeting another. But Mambo has built its entire image on irreverent – though often socially biting – graphics, from its 'farting dog', seen here in one of its many incarnations, through to its ironic captions: 'This bag is made from trees that were blocking ocean views.'

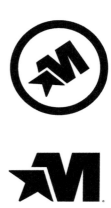

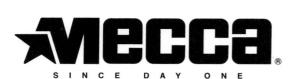

In common with many of the US brands targeting chiefly African-American urban youth, Mecca USA was as much a creation of savvy marketing as of design. After all, this was a brand being worn by the likes of Will Smith on "The Fresh Prince of Bel-Air" and Bill Cosby on "The Cosby Show", not to mention by rapper The Notorious B.I.G. (wearing a 'Chursky' soccer jersey in the video for his debut single "Juicy"), before the name had even been launched at retail. That may have been clever promotion, but it also gave the new brand that did not hail from the grassroots a grassroots appeal beyond the fashion industry salesrooms or the trade shows, such as Magic International in Las Vegas. This was where the label was launched in 1994, backed by Mike Alesko, an early pioneer of the commercial US streetwear market and founder of parent company International News.

International News became a well-known brand in its own right before spawning Mecca, as well as the likes of Alphanumeric (the technical, environmental skatewear brand established in 1998 and counting Forrest Kirby among its sponsored riders), Triko and the influential Seattle store Zebraclub. Indeed, it was two Zebraclub employees, Tony Shellman and fellow salesman Lando Felix, along with their International News boss, Evan Davis, who came up with the idea for Mecca as an aggressively urban clothing company. Alesko (who died in 1998 aged only 59) supported the idea, although differences emerged regarding the direction of Mecca USA. Alesko wanted to expand to create a global lifestyle brand, while the three founders were keen to keep the name low-key and more underground. This led to the latter party selling their interest in 1996 and going on to form Enyce (a phonetic spelling of NYC, although actually pronounced 'eh-nee-chay'), which was later to become a subsidiary of the Italian sportswear giant Fila.

The three founders were perhaps destined for success: two of them, as shop-floor staff, managed to quadruple Zebraclub's Sunday sales by launching an in-store movie matinee club – five dollars bought customers a screening and a five per cent clothing discount. Mecca, meanwhile, rode the wave of the early 1990s urbanwear boom that saw the launch of companies such as Maurice Malone Designs and Karl Kani. In a bid to be considered more as alternative brands rather than ethnic ones, some of these companies sought to transcend the hip-hop-oriented market to join the mainstream, often to find themselves faced with similar corporate wranglings. Karl Kani, for example, was launched in the late 1980s by the designer of the same name, promoted via Los Angeles rap magazines and eventually purchased in 1990 by LA-based Cross Colours, which placed it under its Threads for Life corporate umbrella. By 1993, however, the two companies had parted and Karl Kani Infinity launched in its stead with a dressier attitude.

A sideways step away from the overtly casual or logo-driven is the route Mecca USA also took. Despite its founders' intentions, it did go on to become that all-encompassing label. Its initial collections, aimed at men between 15 and the mid-30s, were expanded to include new lines for children and women. These were promoted as effectively as the menswear, with Mecca Femme being worn by the likes of Queen Latifah, Da Brat and Ananda Lewis. Its product lines, meanwhile, were extended to include not just the brash denim and sweats on which it was founded but more formal styles and more advanced, high-tech fabrications.

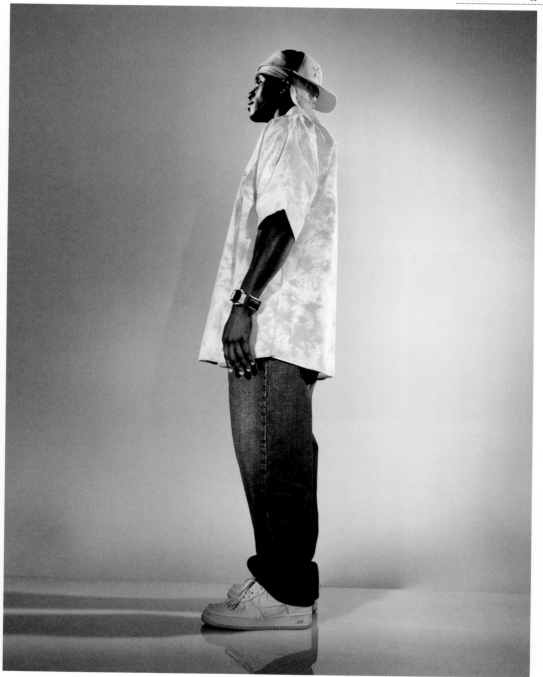

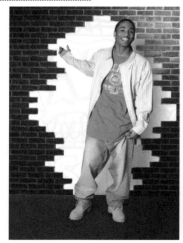
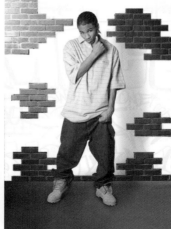
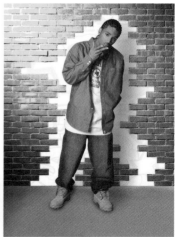

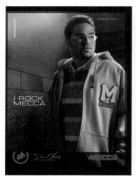
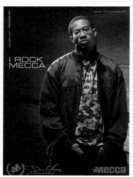
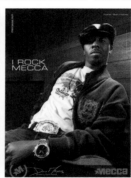
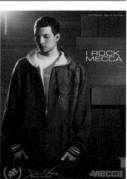

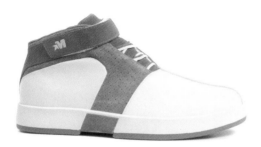
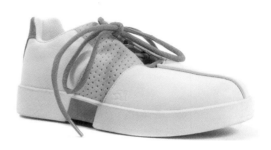

Mecca epitomizes the street style of urban America, which in turn has become the uniform of international youth: the outsize t-shirt and low-slung jeans. The style is said to mimic the way those arrested in the US are forced to wear their trousers once the belt has been confiscated. Mecca has maintained its connection to the streets by using real people rather than models in its advertising.

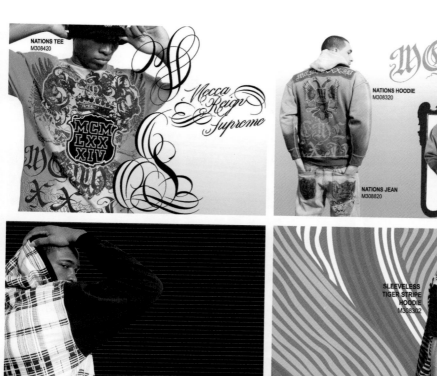

NATIONS TEE
M308420

Mecca Reign Supreme

NATIONS HOODIE
M308320

NATIONS JEAN
M308820

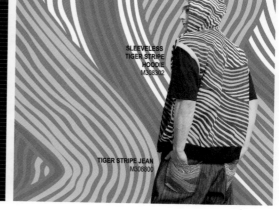

SLEEVELESS
TIGER STRIPE
HOODIE
M308302

TIGER STRIPE JEAN
M308800

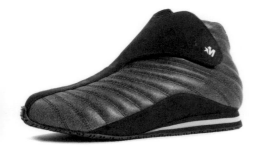

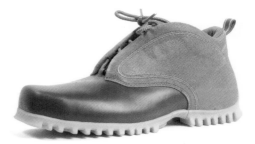

Pages from a Mecca catalogue, as typographically bold as its print designs.

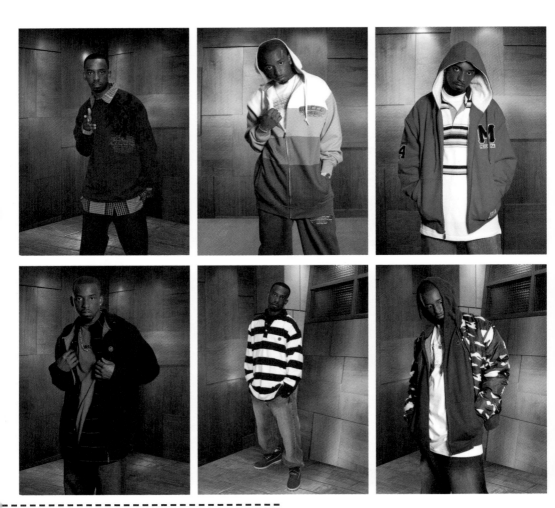

Styles from Mecca's spring/summer 2009 collection, in the studio and, opposite, in
scenes that seem to depict characters in isolation.

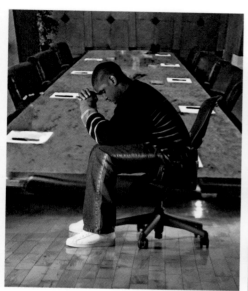

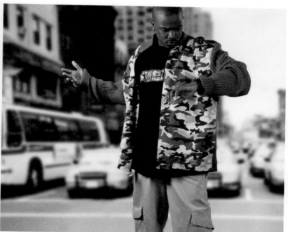

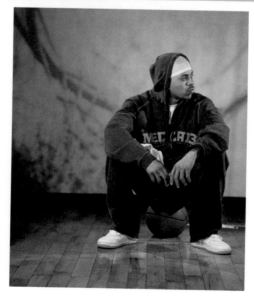

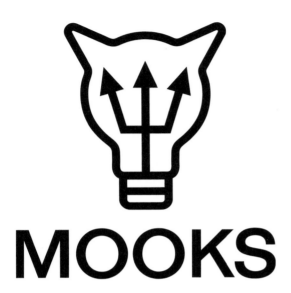

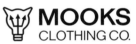

Surfing has certainly always been part of Australian culture, skateboarding less so. But it remains surprising that the country has produced so few streetwear brands of international repute. One exception perhaps, along with Mambo, is Mooks. It was in the late 1980s, in Melbourne, when Peter Hill and his brother Stephen were on the Mambo Easter tour, in the final stages of their pro-skating careers, that they met Richard Allan, who was to change everything for them.

Allan was one of the brains behind the graphic humour of Mambo, the surfwear (and proto-streetwear) label founded in 1984 by surfer Dare Jennings. Allan supported the brothers' idea to launch their own brand as part of their move from skateboarding into building a career in the skateboarding business. This became more concrete as the duo launched Vision Streetwear in Australia. But what financial and investment constraints allowed them to do with it proved limited. "Richard was an advocate of streetwear but thought it could be done better," Peter Hill explained. "He was becoming increasingly frustrated with the beach fashion direction in which his designs were being pushed."

It was over dinner that the brothers decided to go independent and, with Richard Allan on board, launch their own label, provisionally called Moose after Richard Allan's nickname. It was to be a 1970s-inspired brand focusing on simple shapes, denim and sportswear fabrics, targeting an Australian consumer not widely exposed to international brands and, as Peter Hill stated, in a market only just developing its own design community. "Australian design was finally finding its feet after 50 years and the uniquely Australian mix of urban culture located on the coast made the design objective clear. The world has been flooded with rehashed surf fashion and most things post-1970s were tainted with reinterpretation," he said. Moose would look to the past but be purist about it in the process. Or rather, in 1991, when it launched, Mooks would be: why the name was changed from 'Moose' remains uncertain, although 'Mooks' was somehow deemed more credible and interesting, precisely because it was meaningless and abstract.

In fact, the name was borrowed from the script of Martin Scorsese's film *Mean Streets*, in which the question, 'What the fuck is a mook?' is posed. Mook is old New York slang for, depending on the context, a hustler, wiseguy or fool. The original Mooks logo – a freehand design of Richard Allan's – showed touches of Mambo's style but was equally open to interpretation: a lightbulb with a lit element in the shape of a devil's trident. The design was later tidied up and made more symmetrical, in line with the cleaner aesthetic of the brand.

As with Mambo, Allan proved key to shaping the company's artistic direction: designs were based around references to pop art, Japanese manga (comics) and American collegiate sports, and they became a local phenomenon (there were queues around the

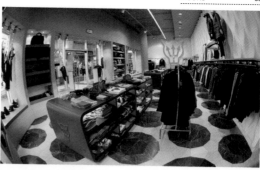

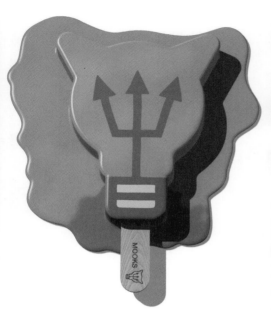

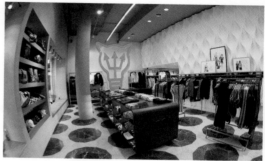

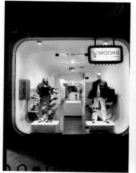

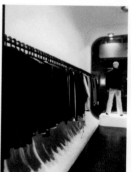

block to the first Mooks store, which opened in Melbourne in 1992) and later a global one. "Richard is an amazing freehand artist and cartoonist," Peter Hill noted. "In fact, Richard is pretty much gifted at everything: patterns, photo direction, fabric knowledge, casting, talent spotting. The only thing he is shit at is claiming credit for what he has done." Allan similarly directed Mooks's early and market-leading black-and-white advertising imagery – shot, as if to emphasize the brand's global ambitions, in downtown Los Angeles – and the subsequent, much-copied graphic silhouette series of colour ads.

This was all part of Mooks's early boom time. In 2000, Allan left the company to take up painting and, having made their money ("We chased the dollar and made some suspect product decisions, probably compromising on chasing the fashion cycle a little," Peter Hill admitted), the brothers sold the company in 2006. Its new owner has since sought to take Mooks back to its more classic roots.

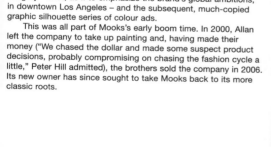

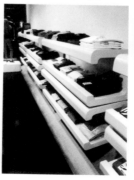

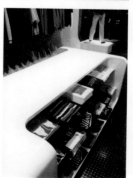

Always among the more modernist and less retro in style, Mooks's clinical, sculptural stores can be akin to the interiors of *2001: A Space Odyssey*.

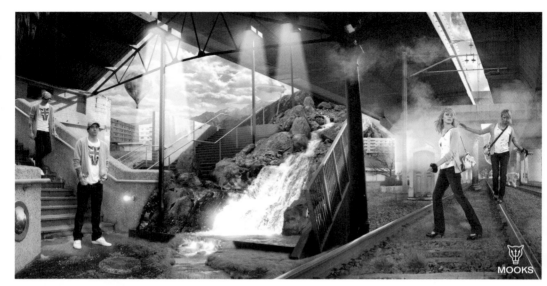

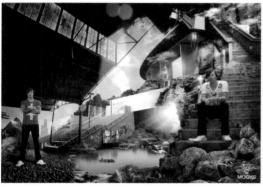

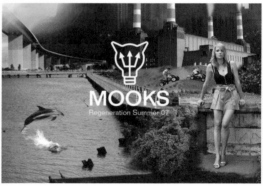

Mooks's advertising campaigns have taken on the sometimes surreal, often satirical tone employed by companies like Diesel – the clothes are secondary to the attitude they embody.

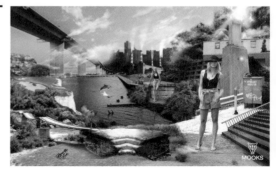

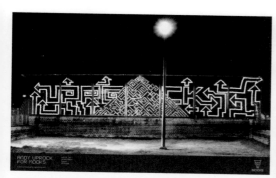

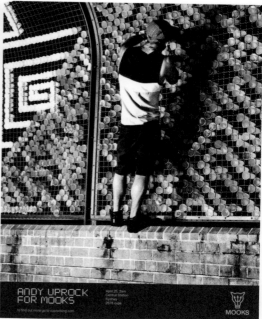

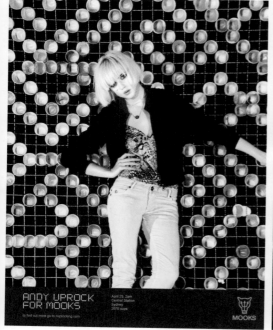

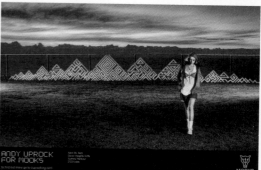

Mooks has worked with Sydney-based B-boy and contemporary artist Andy Uprock, best known for his installation work using plain or brightly coloured cups pressed into the diamond pattern of wire fencing to create patterns or spell out words (he calls it 'cuprocking').

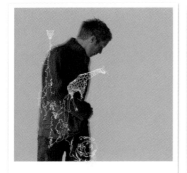
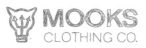

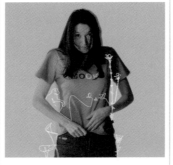
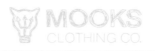

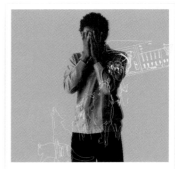
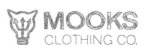

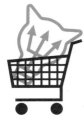

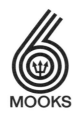
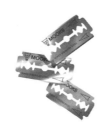

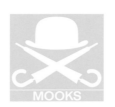
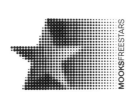

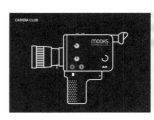
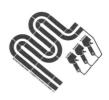

Mooks's graphic logos have taken on a less street and more international flavour,
touching on, among other themes, baseball and stereotypical Britishness, as well
as parodying corporate branding.

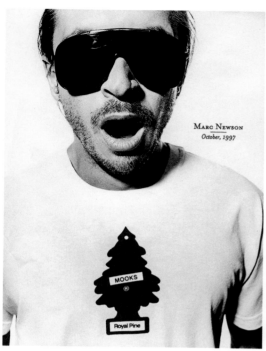

MARC NEWSON
October, 1997

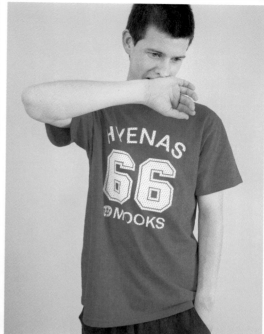

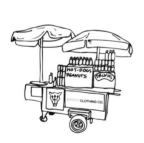

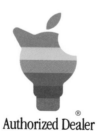

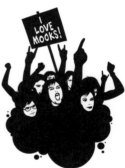

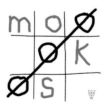

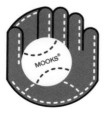

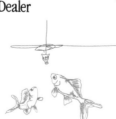

The logos have won the brand a place in Australia's broader design community, including, top left, cross-disciplinary product designer Marc Newson.

NEIGHBORHOOD
TECHNICAL APPAREL®

If military and outdoor clothing have often influenced the design of streetwear, the same cannot be said of motorcycling and cars, albeit very stylish ones. "I am particularly fond of American automobiles from the 1930s and 1940s," says Shinsuke Takizawa, one-time graphic designer and now the man behind Neighborhood. "The few ones I always ride are all in black." Takizawa launched Neighborhood in Tokyo's Harajuku district in 1994, inspired by his passion for motorbikes, cars and the culture that surrounds them. He opened his first Neighborhood shop around the same time as his old friends, Nigo of A Bathing Ape and Jun Takahashi of Undercover, launched their brands. Indeed, the shop was situated near their Nowhere store in Harajuku, so in opening his business he was becoming part of the neighbourhood, a fact which inspired the brand name.

Nigo and Takahashi may be less likely to create the kind of products that have become Takizawa's signature: the leather jacket, technical outerwear, so-called 'damage-processed' denim – with snags, holes and a distinctive asymmetric back pocket – and a more streamlined, almost austere look that brings a sophistication to the baggy t-shirted streetwear stereotypes, all coming together to position Neighborhood as what might be regarded as a thinking man's Von Dutch.

But Takizawa has also built what may at first be regarded as a harder-edged, more masculine style into a lifestyle brand, encompassing film production, accessories, womenswear, childrenswear (introduced in 2006) and homewares, available from a growing number of Hoods, as the brand's stores are referred to. Neighborhood (sometimes shortened to 'NBHD') has even shown at Milan Fashion Week, indicating how it successfully transcends both the underground – including the controversy provoked by a merchandise t-shirt created for the film *Death of a President*, whose graphic expressed the idea of the assassination of President George W. Bush – and the high-fashion markets, for which Takizawa's mechanic-inspired shirts, paint-splattered denims and puffa jackets also work.

So the brand is of high fashion but not really part of it. "Neighborhood is really basic wear, and hence doesn't require a seasonal theme as such. I only want to create clothes with an individual style, the kind I'd like to wear daily," the designer explained. "My taste in music, or in general, hasn't changed since I started studying graphic design. Fashion trends make

little impact on my collections." In fact, Takizawa has suggested that it is precisely because he is of but also slightly outside streetwear, as it is more popularly conceived, that he is able to bring fresh eyes to the many design collaborations with which he has been involved, including those with A Bathing Ape, but also Stussy, Visvim, Supreme New York, Fragment Design and Adidas, for whom he has co-designed. Key to the success of the collaborative product with Adidas was his desire to respect its sporting potential – here, after all, is a global brand whose image is based on making professional sports products – while also being aware that, via Neighborhood, it was likely to be worn on the street. The solution? A very subtle, and oh-so-desirable skull motif embroidered on the heel, and diamond pattern inserts.

Perhaps Takizawa is also put in perspective by his interests – not skating or surfing, neither DJing nor tagging, but custom-building motorbikes, to the level where he has been a competitor in the World and European Championships for Custom Bike-Building. The machines he has presented, such as the Crusader of 2006, are as much works of art as any hand-sculpted and -painted surfboard.

Although most Japanese streetwear designers are too young to remember the US Army's occupation of Japan after the Second World War, the influence of American culture on the Japanese fashion scene remains pervasive, especially in the market for precision reproductions. Neighborhood here (top row) takes its graphic design cue from the personalized embroidery added to the backs of military tour jackets once they were decommissioned.

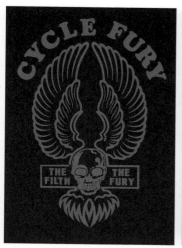

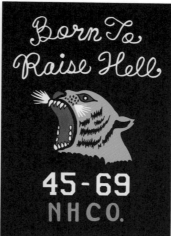

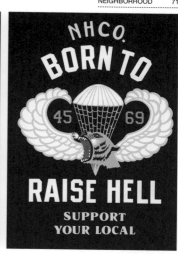

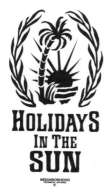

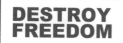

NEIGHBORHOOD

No.3 204

®

TOKYO

NEIGHBORHOOD®TECHNICAL APPAREL
3204, FAF.09 CRAFT WITH PRIDE

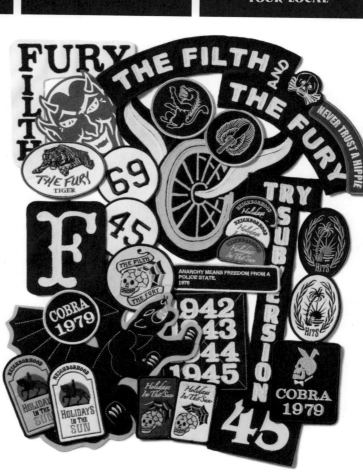

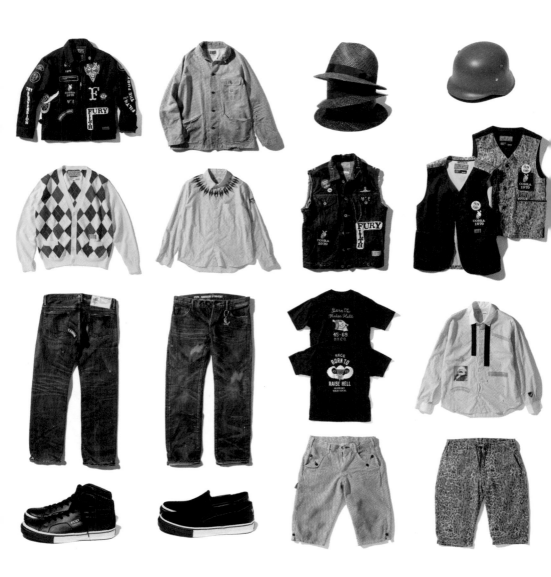

Neighborhood stands apart from streetwear's typical fascination with the skate
and surf scenes. It is drawn more to biker culture, especially that of the 1960s and
1970s: black predominates, silver jewellery is part of the mix, and even the standard-
issue infantry helmet of the German Wehrmacht, a Hell's Angel staple, is reproduced
(top row far right).

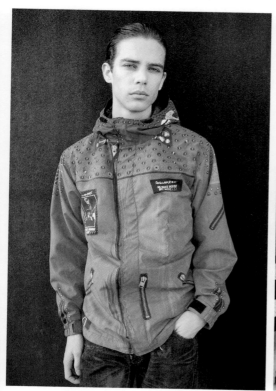

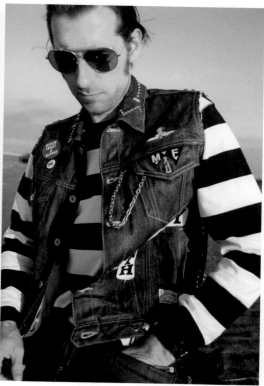

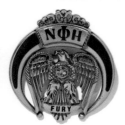

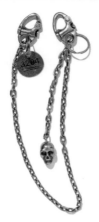

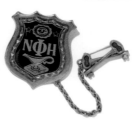

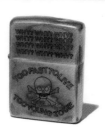

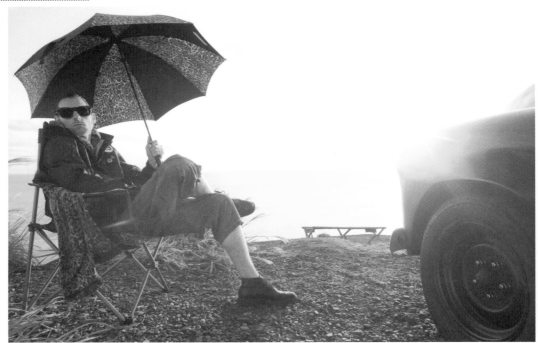

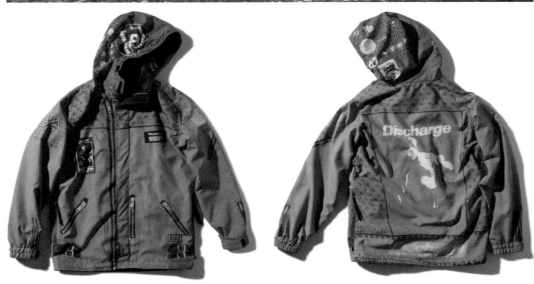

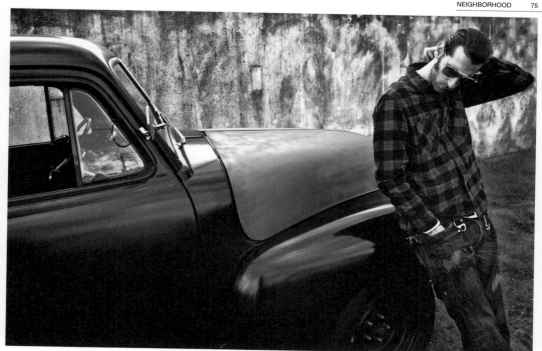

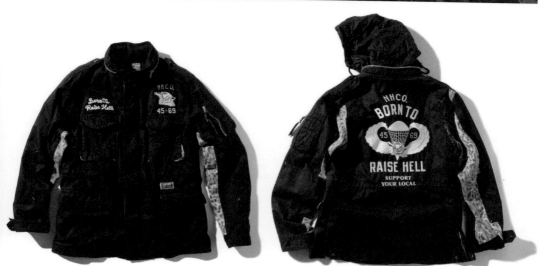

Neighborhood's promotional imagery is timeless, in that it is a blend of the current and the past. The leopard-print umbrella suggests today, but much of the clothing and the car recall the America of the 1950s. For all their apparent simplicity, the jackets are highly technical garments.

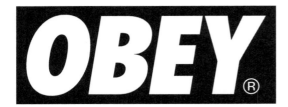

Obey is as much a phenomenon of street art as of clothing. Shepard Fairey began making t-shirts while in high school, spray-painting stencils directly onto blanks, with the graphics mostly punk-band-related. But one renegade image, knocked up in five minutes in the back of a coffee shop, captured his imagination: that of the late André Roussimoff, aka André the Giant, a famed wrestler. By 1989 Fairey was studying illustration at the Rhode Island School of Design and learning to screenprint, putting his t-shirts onto a more commercial footing.

By then, the dark, glaring eyes of his Orwellian André icon – all bold black and white and sometimes immensely tall and wide – and the challenging, accompanying buzzword 'Obey', had spread far and wide. This was almost because of, rather than in spite of, the image being essentially meaning-free; but it was also thanks to some hard graft and extensive travelling that saw Fairey sticker, wheat-paste and stencil it as far afield as Boston and Philadelphia (and since then onto the streets of the UK, Japan, Australia and Singapore – getting Fairey jailed for vandalism in five cities along the way, and arrested for "advertising without a permit"). Inspired by the work of LA-based postermaker Robbie Conal during the late 1980s, Fairey reclaimed billboards from the corporate world, which used its financial might to infest the streets with unwanted persuasions to spend.

That alone was a stunning case study of what Fairey referred to, perhaps in an attempt to legitimize his illegal activities, as "an experiment in phenomenology. I don't think it's great art. It's an act of perseverance. It was an experiment in how far you can take an absurd idea using all the devices of advertising and propaganda used to infiltrate a society," he said. "Just planting something out there that's provocative and not explained and is all over the place, it does something. I really thought that it was something nobody had exploited to its full potential outside the realm of advertising and on a much more insidious, grassroots level that wasn't some sort of religion or cult. My thing's been called all of those things."

In other words, just how far could a graphic, without clear content, tap reflexively into the public consciousness? How would a branding campaign with no product succeed? It certainly provided a logo with a credibility that many brands would kill for; and when a product did follow, it had a ready market from day one. Yet, chiefly for Fairey, t-shirts and skateboards, as much as billboards, lampposts and the sides of buildings, have become just another medium for pop-culture references – count among them Kiss, Marilyn Monroe, Jesse Jackson, Jimi Hendrix and Slayer, as

well as takes on the historic propaganda of Mao and Lenin, celebrity deconstruction and Fairey's own, often humanitarian, political commentary. As he put it: "If somebody just donated a billboard to me, a lot of graffiti guys would say, 'Dude, that's legal, so it ain't real.' But for me, it's about the exposure, not whether it's legal or illegal."

So, one can only imagine how pleased Fairey must be with the countless thousands of André/Obey t-shirts that have now sold. Fans become walking billboards, as they have for the many other street artists whose work has found itself becoming an apparel line (or found on rugs, pillowcases or toys); notably, that of Lenny McGurr and Josh Franklin, better known as the graffiti writers Futura and Stash (trading also under the Recon name). It wasn't until 2001 that Obey Clothing (with the assistance of graphic artists Mike Ternosky and Erin Wignall) made an official launch – that in-built credibility giving it a pulling power that would see it collaborate with rappers such as Public Enemy, whose own famed target logo was reworked for a special collection.

Meanwhile, Fairey established himself as less the streetwear entrepreneur and more the hit and legit graphic artist, his work receiving the plaudits of international one-man shows, his Black Market and Studio Number One agencies hired by the likes of Adidas, Led Zeppelin, Airwalk, Universal Pictures, Hasbro Toys and Pepsi (whose billboards Fairey once regularly 'bombed' – "the world is full of contradictions," he noted). This is the corporate world seeking to capture the power of underground imagery, of what was once just the art-student joke, now transformed into a neo-pop-art phenomenon and finally realized as a streetwear leader.

Shepard Fairey at work (opposite top left), postering an alleyway with one of his iconic designs. The stark stencil face is perhaps his most famous work – and made the easy transition from wall to chest.

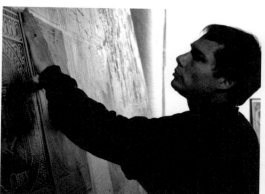

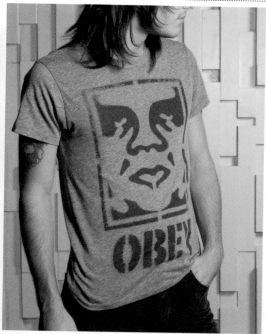

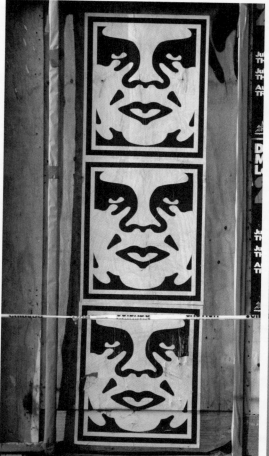

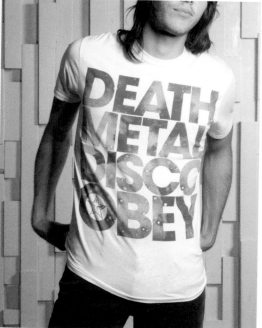

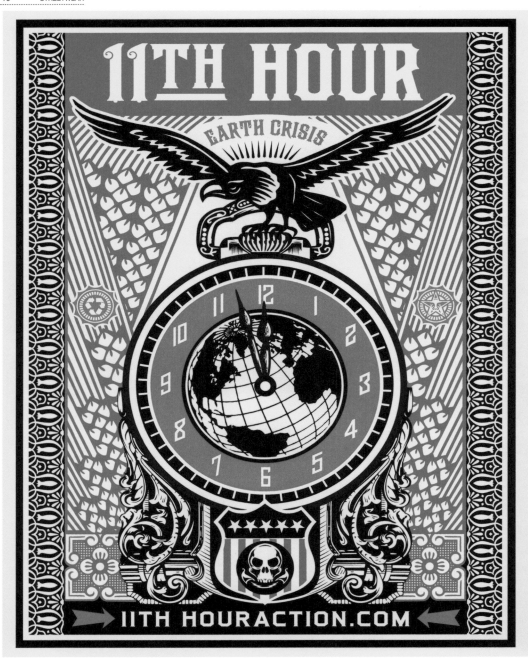

Fairey's charity t-shirt design for the 11th Hour Action Network, a community working for a more sustainable society and sharing ideas about green living – a more direct example of the socio-political stance of much of Fairey's work.

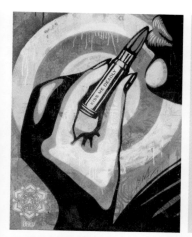

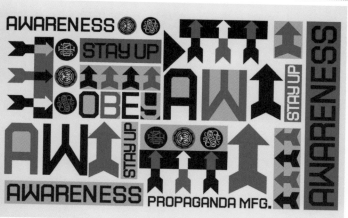

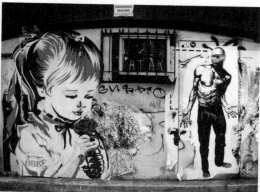

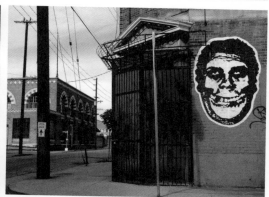

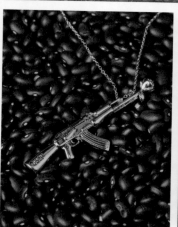

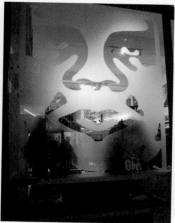

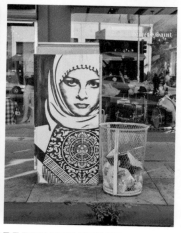

Fairey's work was born on the street, but it has proven just as effective in other media, be they prints, shop windows or pieces of jewellery. The rose in the barrel of an AK-47 assault rifle is an updated reference to anti-Vietnam War protests of the 1960s and 1970s.

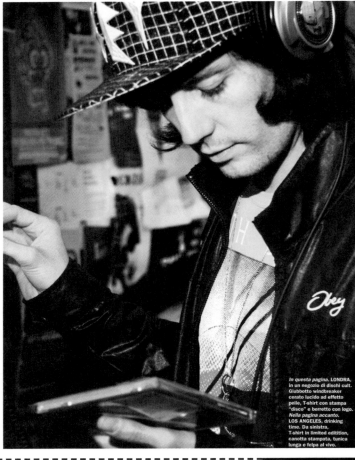

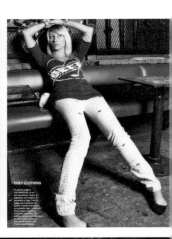

In questa pagina, LONDRA, in un negozio di dischi cult. Giubbotto windbreaker cerato lucido ad effetto pelle, T-shirt con stampa "disco" e berretto con logo. Nella pagina accanto, LOS ANGELES, drinking time. Da sinistra, T-shirt in limited editition, canotta stampata, tunica lunga e felpa al vivo.

OBEY CLOTHING

Can Fairey's work straddle both the commercial and the political? Naysayers have suggested that to attempt to do so is to sell out. But Fairey has managed to build a fashion business from his graphics and phrases without limiting his artistic commentary on current affairs, as with the Barack Obama print opposite.

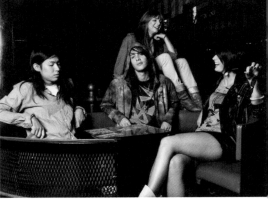

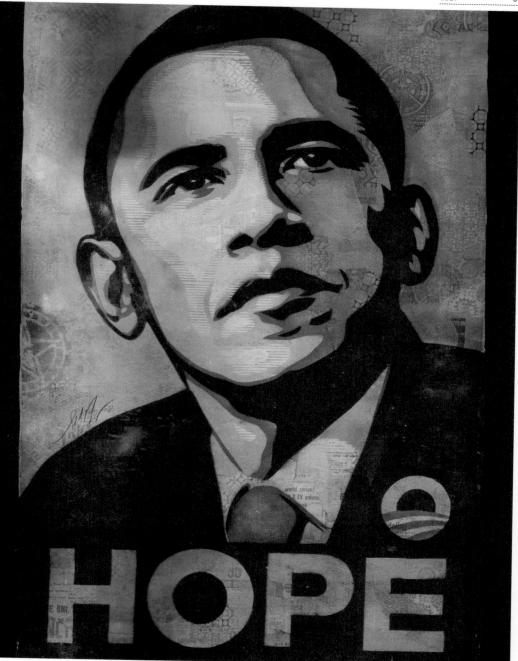

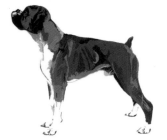
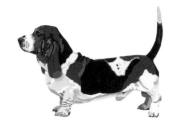
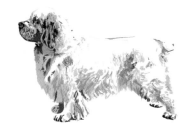

ONETrueSaxon®

As a marketing strategy, it was certainly a bold one. When British streetwear label One True Saxon launched in the UK, it proclaimed that it was "only available in the North". The trio that founded the brand in 1998, Ian Bergin, Mark Bailey and Ian Paley – all ex-employees of the fashion brand Paul Smith, with Paley the brand's jeanswear designer – had grown tired of fashion's overly close associations with London, at the expense of a vibrant, more underground scene in the north of the country. Their answer? The Nottingham-based One True Saxon's graphic-printed t-shirts, sweatshirts, nylon jackets and Japanese denim – much of it carrying the brand's Staffordshire bull terrier logo – would not be available south of the Watford Gap, which has unofficially denoted a north–south divide ever since the first UK motorway was built.

Similarly, the label's retrospective prints and patterns stemmed from the references of a shared northern upbringing, but quickly appealed to diverse streetwear groups: skaters as well as northern 'terrace casuals'. It grew out of a certain passion for subcultures found more readily in the north of the UK – "that was the difference between the north and the south back then: in the north there was not as much scope [in fashion] so everyone frenzied on the few things that were available," Paley explained. And with talk of "the toff influence" of the south and its "complacent" fashion buyers, unwilling to source the new or adventurous, the brand came loaded with an appealing edge.

That said, One True Saxon had substance behind the fighting talk. It helped (as the 'Saxon' component of its name might suggest) foster the notion that a streetwear brand could hail from the UK, rather than, as is more typical, the US or Japan. Collaboration with fellow British streetwear brand Addict cemented this idea. In a nod to the ape-shaped camouflage designs of A Bathing Ape, together the companies created a special camo design that integrated the One True Saxon dog logo to the extent that the outline was effectively camouflaged itself, and later co-designed heavyweight graphic-printed sweats. Other collaborations have included those with British 'Monsterism' graphic designer Pete Fowler.

"The notion of a British streetwear brand usually ends up going one way – history has dictated the route well: aspire to the rich," Paley said. "What we wanted to achieve was something that was influenced by all aspects of British culture, whether it be good or bad. Saxon has its roots in people, in conversations over a pint, the humour in the everydayness of being British." The brand has managed, however, to avoid being too parochial: in 2002, for example, it collaborated with New York street art collective Faile and Bast to use their artwork as linings to limited-edition jeans and field jackets.

One True Saxon also, alongside streetwear brands and retailers such as Supreme in the US and Neighborhood in Japan, helped to develop a more sophisticated, details-driven take on streetwear – clothing that young skaters could, in effect, graduate to once oversized tops and combats no longer seemed appropriate. As Paley once noted emphatically, "We are not a big baggy skate label producing crap, low-quality tees." It was to this end that One True Saxon was, for example, in 2003 able to join forces with the southern Chinese hand-crafted denim specialists Indigo Farm to produce a range of jeans limited to just 100 pairs. Each pair sold for a four-figure sum.

Indeed, it was not without reason that One True Saxon's mission statement was taken from *Modern Manners and Social Forms*, a 19th-century manual on dress etiquette: "Don't dress like a 'dude' or a 'swell', nor carry a little poodle dog (a man's glory is his strength and manliness – not in aping silly girls), nor cock your hat on one side, nor tip it back on your head (let it sit straight and square), nor wear anything conspicuous or that will make you offensive to others."

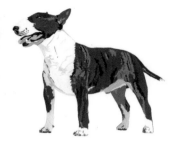
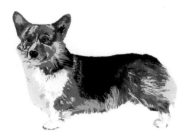
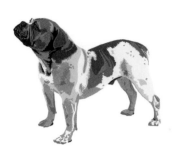

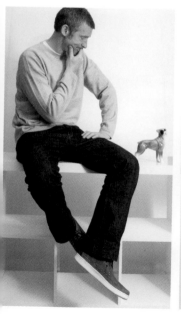
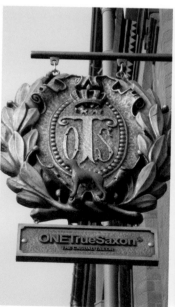
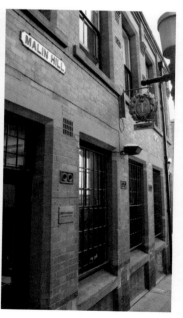

Dogs have always played a part in One True Saxon's graphic world, not least the boxer dog, far left, which was adopted as the brand's main logo, seen on the sign outside of its offices in Nottingham, England and, overleaf, even worked into a camouflage design. Above left, Ian Bergin, managing director of the brand.

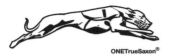

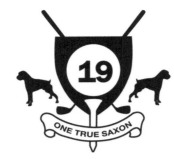

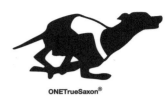

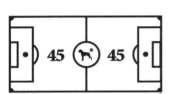

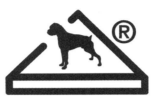

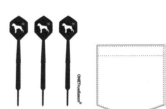

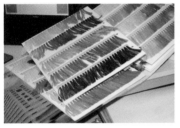

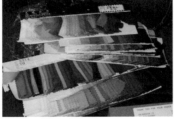

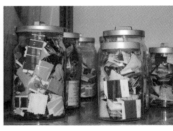

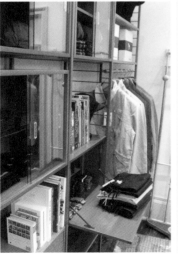

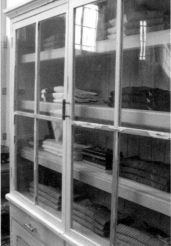

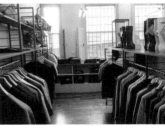

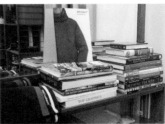

The iconography used by One True Saxon in its various logos has always played less with skate and surf than with British sporting archetypes: greyhound racing, golf, darts, snooker and soccer. Samples, swatches, mood boards and inspirational books around the One True Saxon offices all feed into the company's designs.

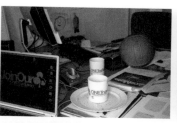
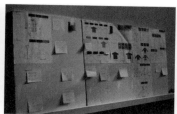
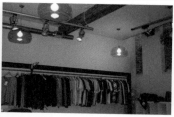
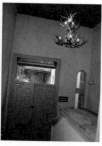
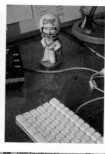
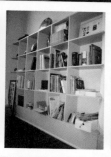
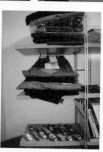
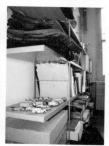

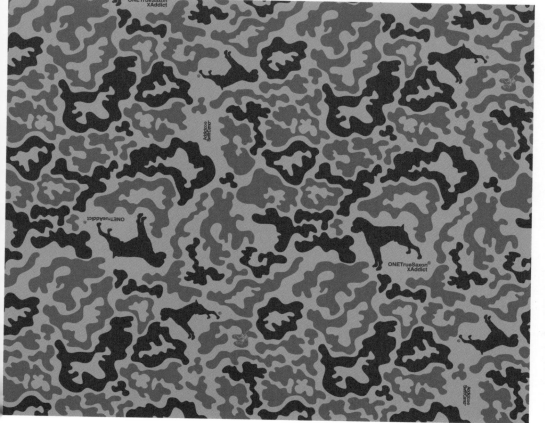

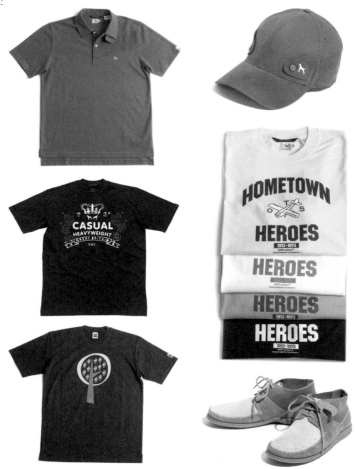

One True Saxon's strength has always been the purity and simplicity of its design, which touches on streetwear traditions without being enveloped by them: their styles consequently lean towards the plain and timeless, such as the classic polo shirt opposite.

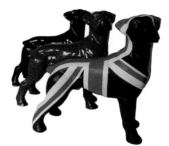

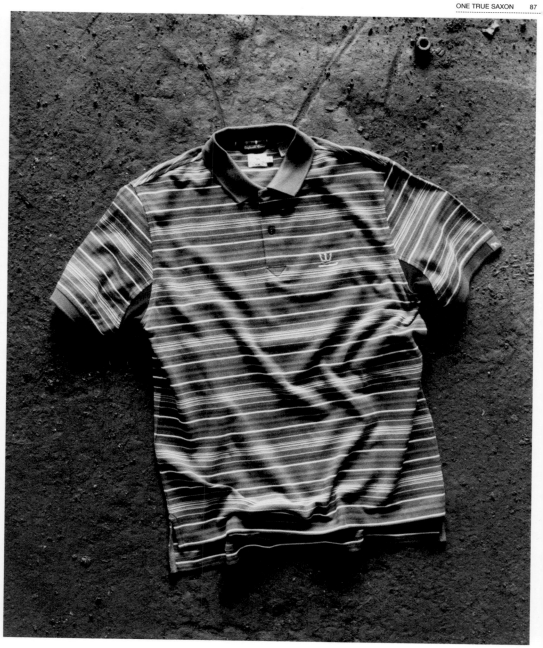

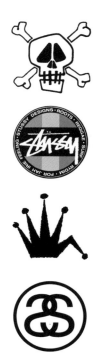

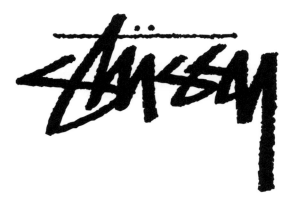

When the surfer met Frank Sinatra while skiing, who could predict that the relationship would grow into a hugely influential streetwear label? The surfer, though, was one Shawn Stussy and Sinatra – not *the* Sinatra, of course – was his business partner. It all began at the crest of 1980 at Newport Beach, in southern California, where Stussy was a 'shaper', making surfboards that became instantly recognizable throughout the US surf scene. His boards, with flat decks and a beaked nose, were distinctive. What was written on them was even more so. Each was airbrushed and scribbled with Stussy's Continental, double-dotted, Germanic signature (in homage to his Austrian-German ancestry) that would come to grace the clothing line, referencing graffiti tagging but also the logo culture of international branding. That signature evolved over the years and is now acknowledged globally. The company talks of the "original stock" and the "graffiti stock", in reference to early and later versions of the signature, with Shawn Stussy always using a Sharpie pen to write it, even on cheques.

Although Stussy had no formal fashion training, his mother and sister were seamstresses, so he knew his way around fabric, thread and needle. Together with a stint designing graphics for early surf label Gotcha, he had the two skills to start with home-made caps and t-shirts, selling out from the trunk of his car to the Laguna Beach crowd. Sinatra's entrepreneurial input built the beginnings of a brand that, while born in streetwear, superseded it, came from the underground but took streetwear overground.

That early hip-hop and the LA punk scenes were king perhaps meant the world was not quite ready for a full clothing line that would pioneer the graphic t-shirt – not to mention popularize cargo trousers, chain wallets, outsized shirts, mix military with preppy and surf influences and launch a million me-toos. But that would surely follow, as wipeout follows rogue wave. After all, Stussy was helping to create a new dress aesthetic: taking the influences of the edgier music genres of the time, crossbreeding them with the graphic qualities of street art, but also pop art and New York's neo-expressionism, and then splicing those with the sartorial touches not just of surf and skate style but functional military and workwear garments.

It was the same style and substance philosophy applied to Stussy's boards: meticulously crafted but also bearing a distinctive graphic gloss. And, although there were other companies selling to the surfers and skaters before it, among them the likes of Quiksilver and OP, Jimmy'Z and Powell, Stussy can probably lay claim to being the progenitor brand of modern streetwear.

Inevitably, by the time surf and skateboard culture took off, Stussy was waiting to cater to some of the leading skaters of the day, from Keith Hufnagel to Anthony Van Engelen. A Stussy skate team was born. The company cleverly maintained an underground status while pushing itself more as a lifestyle brand than as a purveyor of clothes for a then niche activity, and the makings of a globally popular look were set in stone. Or put on wheels.

Shawn Stussy may have bowed out of the business, selling his share about a decade ago, but by then his namesake brand was well on its way to becoming a multi-million-dollar monolith, worn in their time by everyone from Madonna to Public Enemy,

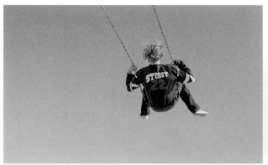
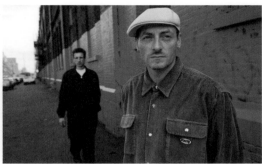
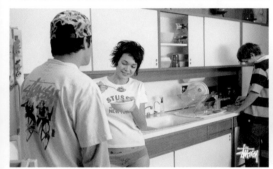
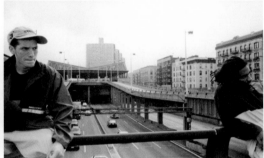

with a fanatical following in Japan and stores from New York to London, Milan to Bali. Well, have surfboard, will travel. Perhaps simply due to its longevity, the brand has also notched up more collaborations – the marketing benchmark of the successful streetwear brand – than any other company in the streetwear market; among them with Burton Snowboards, Nike (for which it designed a take on the sports giant's iconic Dunks sneakers) and the Commonwealth t-shirt label.

It also followed its younger fans as they have grown older in launching a Deluxe line of clothing – dressier without dismissing the workwear aesthetic entirely, and made from luxury fabrics such as chambray, poplin and Japanese twill. Stussy, in fact, is fortunate enough to have a committed and global fan base that has ensured its longevity. The Stussy take on streetwear has helped transform it from a product aimed initially at youth culture to a more sophisticated one embraced by those for whom youth is a distant memory, from what the company has described as being "from classic street to luxury street". It also enabled Stussy to be regarded, as it always intended, more as a lifestyle than a skate label.

Indeed, there are those who suggest that, in growing, Stussy has lost its original anti-establishment edge. Take, for example, its graphic tees' one-time take on the hip-hop 'sampling' principle: appropriations of high-fashion labels from Gucci (reworked as Stucci) to Louis Vuitton and Chanel. Yet the company has since also sued graphic designer, pop iconography-reworker and Freshjive founder Rick Klotz for doing the same with the Stussy logo. Facing accusations of selling out is perhaps inevitable for any brand that launches in an act of rebellion but also wants to be of international significance. Not without reason did Sinatra once say that Shawn Stussy "always wanted to be like Armani". Still, far from being the Gap of urban streetwear, Stussy's historic status as a trendsetter par excellence remains.

The original Stussy logo, above left, hand-written by founder Shawn Stussy, the Germanic umlaut added for visual effect rather than grammar. Note the double-S logo, a neat take on the double-C logo of French couture house Chanel. Above: Stussy advertising shots from the 1990s.

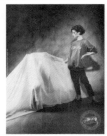
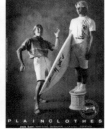
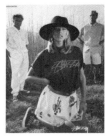
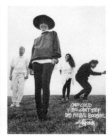
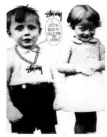
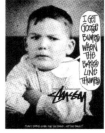
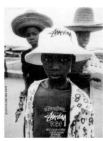
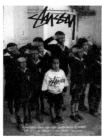

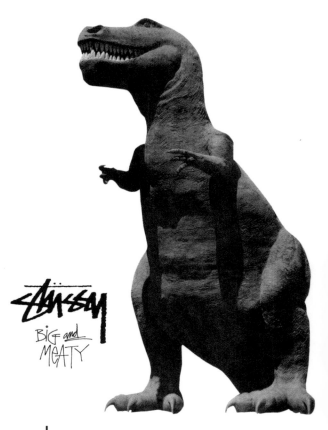

As a pioneer, Stussy's early advertising imagery did not fall into the trap of streetwear cliché, but rather played with all forms, from traditional fashion plate to snapshot, humour to found imagery, often not showing the product at all. Surrealism also became a tool – hence the dinosaur.

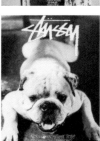
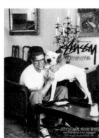
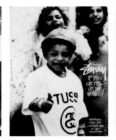
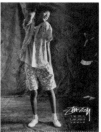
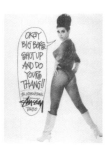

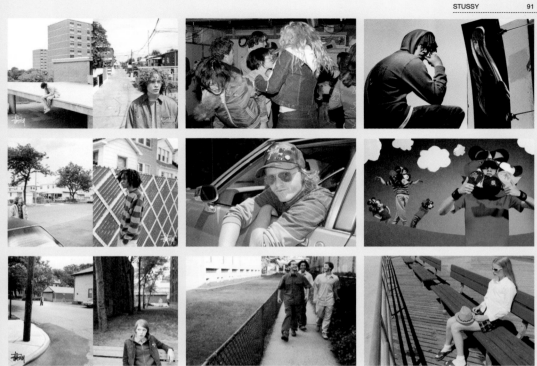

Ad campaigns of the 1990s and beyond have reflected diverse moods, from the whimsical to (in the centre panels) a vérité style shot by photographer Terry Richardson. Graphics, such as those below, have been equally diverse, with a penchant for Rodchenko-style montage.

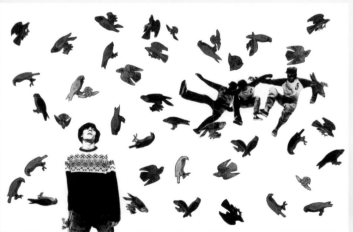

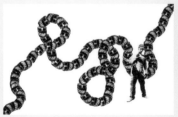

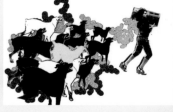

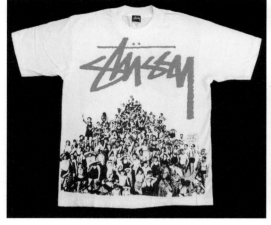

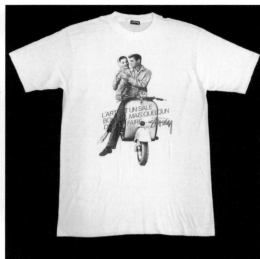

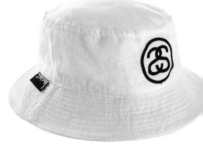

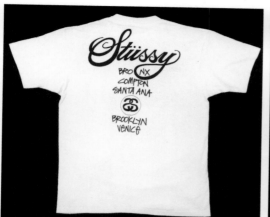

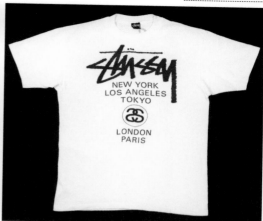

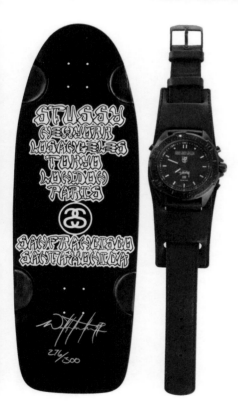

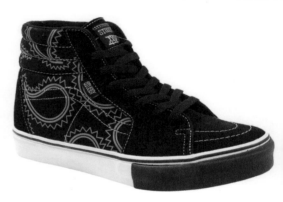

Stussy has become a brand with sufficient potency to lend its name to diverse products, from watches to wakeboards, monographs to casual womenswear. But it has always stayed close to its roots: one t-shirt may list the traditional fashion capitals but another cites Stussy's own West and East Coast versions: Bronx, Compton, Santa Ana, Brooklyn, Venice.

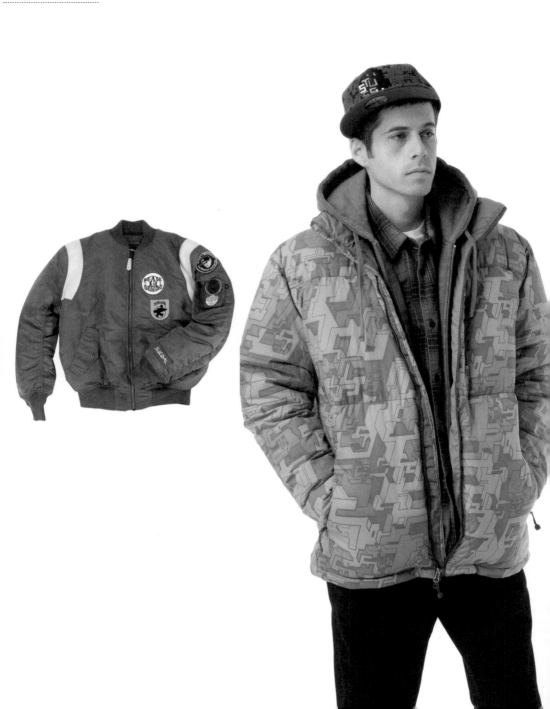

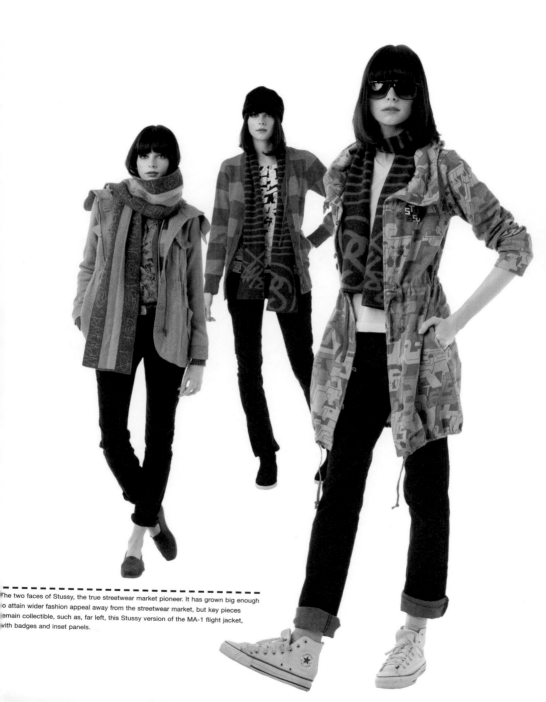

The two faces of Stussy, the true streetwear market pioneer. It has grown big enough to attain wider fashion appeal away from the streetwear market, but key pieces remain collectible, such as, far left, this Stussy version of the MA-1 flight jacket, with badges and inset panels.

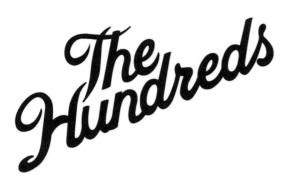

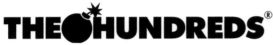

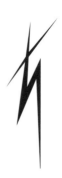

When, in his early twenties, Bobby Kim set up The Hundreds with friend Ben Shenassafar, not even he could have predicted how quickly their company would take off. One of three children of Korean immigrants, Kim grew up in multicultural Los Angeles and, inevitably, took to the West Coast surf, skate and hip-hop scenes. It is perhaps a sign of how far grassroots movements have grown up and become serious enterprises that he and Shenassafar – the child of Iranian immigrants – met not at the skatepark, but in the first-year classes of law school, seeking to fulfil parental wishes that they become respectable professionals. They bonded over a mutual interest in art and design and, while later both half-heartedly took their bar exams ("law school strips you of all your creativity," Kim warned), law inevitably began to take a back seat. Indeed, the duo had long had it in mind to go into business regardless. In its stead was the plan, launched with $400, to design and make t-shirts under the name of The Hundreds.

"Saying that something is happening by the hundreds connotes a great deal of force," Kim explained. "There's energy and strength in numbers. The less sexy answer is that I was playing around with the typography and the letters looked cool."

The graphics they design are referential in ways less obviously cool than many (more nostalgia-obsessed) streetwear brands, but all the more cool for that: quotes from the film *Willy Wonka and the Chocolate Factory* and images from *Peter Pan* have featured. The last is appropriate: when it became clear that law would not be the duo's future, but with t-shirt orders in the thousands, Kim noted that "we never have to grow up". Yet from the outset the pair have worked with the attitude that bigger, older, more

groundbreaking streetwear names came to adopt over time, as they built the market The Hundreds now shares with them.

"There are 50 new t-shirt lines that come out every day," Kim pointed out. "We really emphasized that we weren't a t-shirt line – we were more lifestyle. We aimed to bring this subculture out. It's just the idea of trying to be rebellious. Or trying to be a little bit anti, questioning government or your parents, trying to do something different. I feel like these kids – all they know is sneaker-collecting and buying t-shirts, and they don't think about anything else. Every t-shirt brand is just something stupid – a rapper and some guns. I'd like [The Hundreds] to say something." A phrase on one of their t-shirts, 'The strong take from the weak, but the smart take from the strong', might serve as a mantra.

The Hundreds may not claim to be a pioneer, to have been there at the very beginning. But it is representative of a new millennial wave of small brands – such as, among many others, 10.Deep, King Stampede, Crooks & Castles – that are reshaping streetwear culture into the more underground phenomenon it was originally. Kim has denounced the "commercialized" takes on the streetwear market as a "big-industry ruse" and insisted on a limited, specialist distribution for the brand. "The essence of streetwear is that you don't want to look like everybody else," he noted. "When people ask them, 'Hey, where did you get that?', they want to say, 'Oh, you don't know? Well, you can't get one. Good luck on eBay'."

For all its exclusivity, The Hundreds is also one of the fastest-growing new generation brands and has certainly been busy since it launched in 2003. There is the clothing, its design ethos being to echo the surf style of the 1980s and the independent

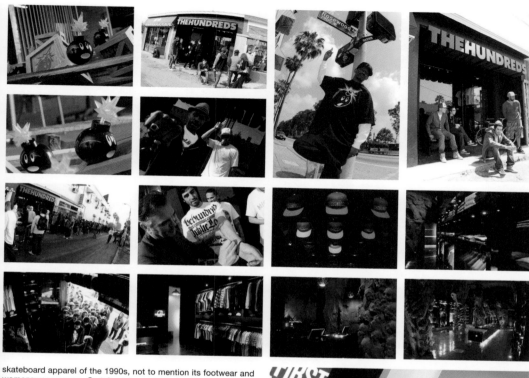

skateboard apparel of the 1990s, not to mention its footwear and womenswear ranges. Certain styles, notably its all-over paisley-print hoodies, have sold out within hours, only to receive that backhanded compliment of being found for sale, yes, on eBay at three times their retail price. And it can count among its collaborative projects those with Gravis, Casio, Disney and Es, among others.

The Hundreds' blog is also a serious street culture portal rather than random ramblings, a product of Kim having majored in media and communications and worked for a spell on the editorial team of a San Diego-based, internationally distributed youth culture magazine. Even his parents have been satisfied: one of his brothers became a lawyer.

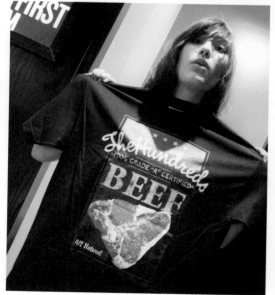

The Hundreds store in LA has become as much a cultural and community hub as a place to shop, drawing huge queues – as well as Morrissey – to some events and product launches.

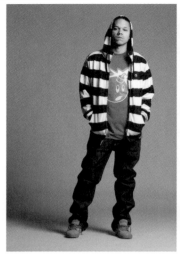
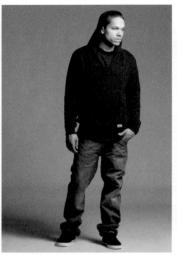
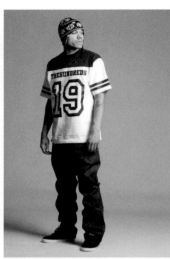

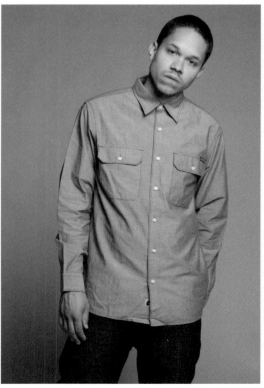
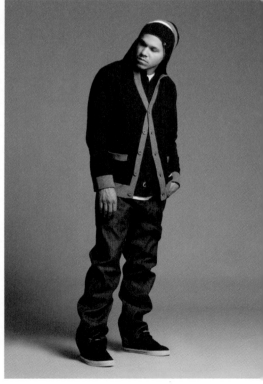

Rather than ape the standard outsized streetwear style of the American West Coast, as a younger brand The Hundreds has pursued a cleaner, at times preppyish aesthetic, as strong in shirts, for example, as in t-shirts.

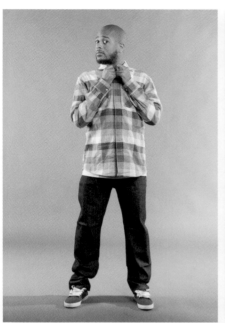
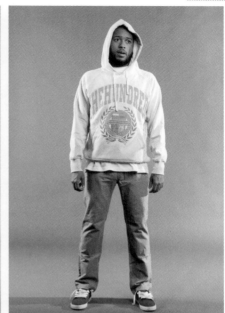
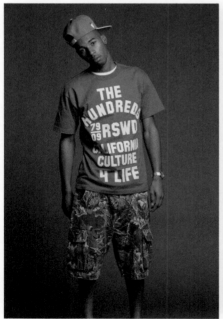
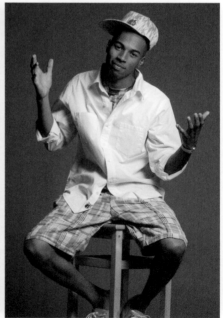

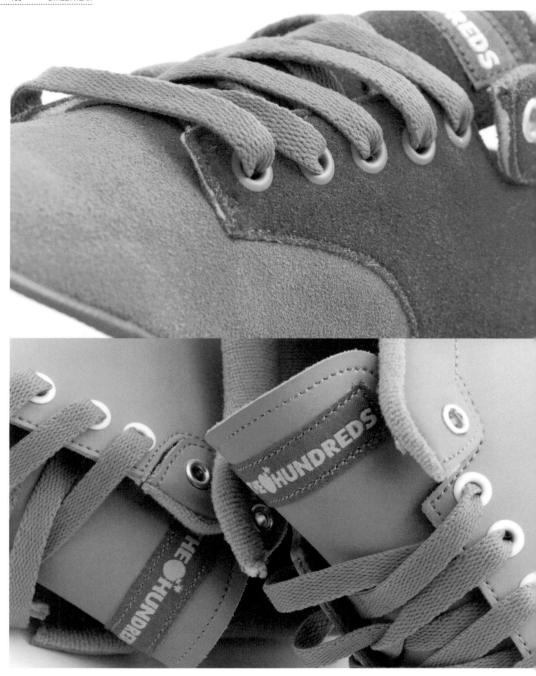

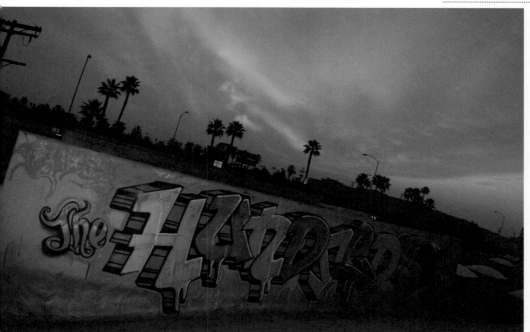

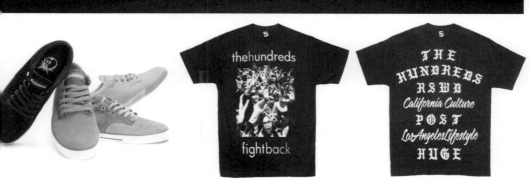

neakers have become one of The Hundreds' particular strengths. They choose to
esign their own styles – often with a distinctive colour palette – rather than work
collaboration with established sports footwear brands.

triple five *Soul*

"The whole early 1990s in New York saw a lot of organic growth in business. I just happened to live in a store-front apartment, with a sewing machine in the store and my apartment in the back," the founder of Triple Five Soul, Camella Ehlke, said. "I started buying miscellaneous fabrics and started making things for me and my friends. To see someone I didn't know in something we made was like, 'Oh my god!'"

"If you ask me why streetwear, why all these hip-hop clothes, it was just a question of pursuing one's own style. A lot of my friends were in the music industry, streetwear was getting sporty and hip-hop was at a pivotal moment – a very mixed, downtown culture and a lot of fun. There was no big business plan. Even the logo was an accident – a graphic designer [Alyasha Owerka-Moore] who was just this skater dude designed some logos in exchange for a couple of hats. It's much harder now [to launch a business] and survive. Back then a lot of people told me to give it up when it got hard. But it was my baby."

Ehlke herself no longer works with the brand she established in 1989 when she was just 19 and an art and design student at New York's Pratt University. She left the company in 2003 to launch a modern bed-and-breakfast establishment in upstate New York with her chef husband. But when she launched her label – then a streetwear brand that designed its own fabrics, evoking surfwear and bohemian, retro styles back to the 1960s, from hoodies to velour suits, all with a home-made quality – she broke new ground. This was not least for being the only pioneering streetwear company established solo by a woman, but for establishing a brand that grew up as part of the community it served; thus, if only accidentally, becoming a business role model for many other streetwear brands with grassroots heritage.

Triple Five Soul (sometimes also known as 555 Soul) was "a whole urban lifestyle – a movement of artists, musicians, dancers and DJs," Ehlke said. This has meant counting Mos Def among her friends (he was the face of Triple Five Soul's first advertising campaign, and the brand designed a special line for the rapper/ actor), building close ties with local art scenes – including World Music Conference sponsorship and the funding of *Scratch*, the first full-length documentary on turntablism. The Ludlow Street store, the company's first, was a hangout – with dancehall parties run out of the store's backyard and underground mix tapes sold by the cash register – but despite this, the company's wares quickly developed a cult following in Japan. Even the company name was haphazard, a tongue-in-cheek reference to one of the telephone party lines then advertised across the city's Lower East Side.

The company's growth was also somewhat random. One of Ehlke's distinctive tie hats was spotted on MTV, sported by hip-hop historian and graffiti writer Fab 5 Freddy, driving a flood of customers to her store. But the brand really took off in 1997, after production was more professionally handled (in exchange for 50 per cent of the business) by Troy Morehouse, an ex-licensed manufacturer for Phat Farm. The shift up in gears also saw Triple Five Soul win a reputation for offering not just collectible streetwear items – such as its wool cargo pants, anti-George W. Bush t-shirts, the 5 Deadly Venoms t-shirt designed by SSUR's Russell K, or those by graffiti artist Stash – but functional items too, including a backpack whose frame detaches to create a chair and a DJ case with in-built wheels. Despite Triple Five Soul now being a multi-million-dollar brand, it has kept a ceiling on its growth through tight distribution, expanding the business through the launch of more mass-market, spin-off labels such as Subscript

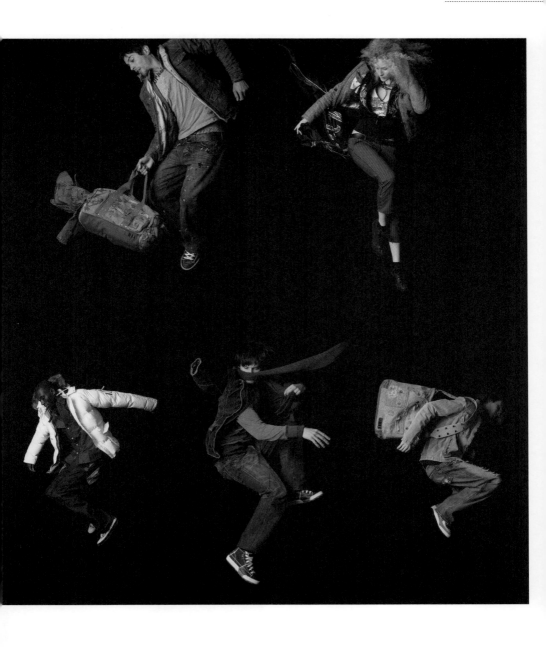

Triple Five Soul's energized, mostly clean-cut image has allowed it to transcend the standard streetwear market, appealing to women as much as men.

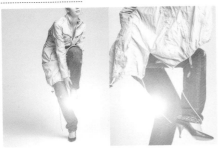
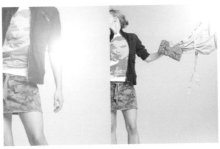
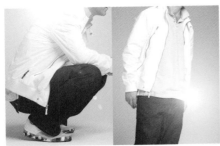
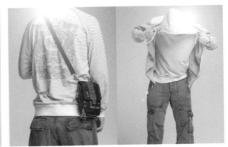
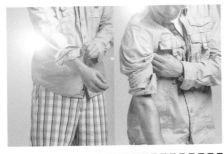

Rather than playing on the clichéd urban images of the streetwear market, Triple Five Soul has embraced an upbeat tempo as a lifestyle brand with more mainstream fashion leanings. Its advertising imagery (opposite top two rows) has, nevertheless, occasionally been brooding and esoteric.

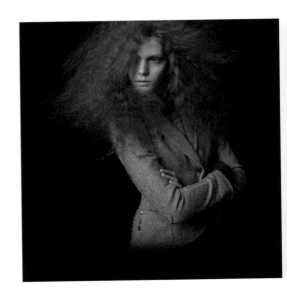

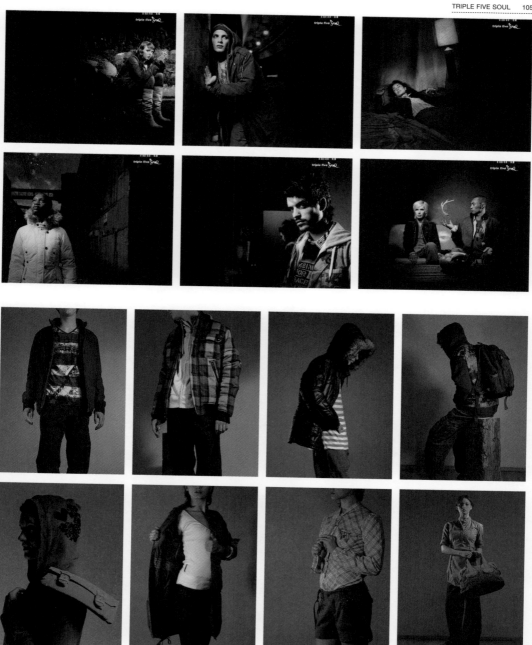

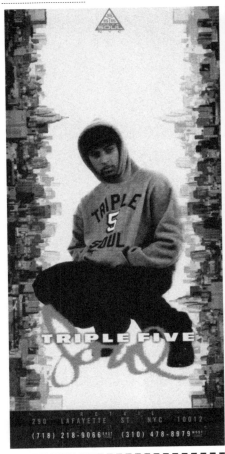

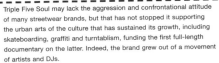

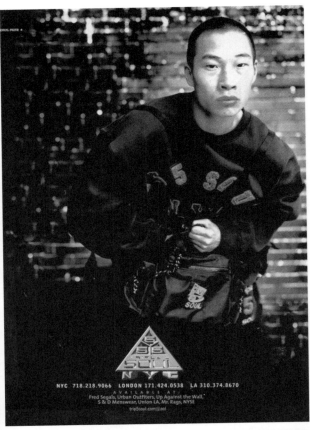

Triple Five Soul may lack the aggression and confrontational attitude of many streetwear brands, but that has not stopped it supporting the urban arts of the culture that has sustained its growth, including skateboarding, graffiti and turntablism, funding the first full-length documentary on the latter. Indeed, the brand grew out of a movement of artists and DJs.

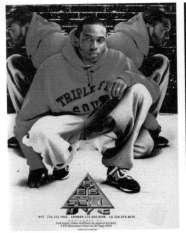

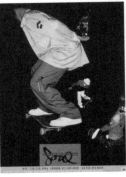

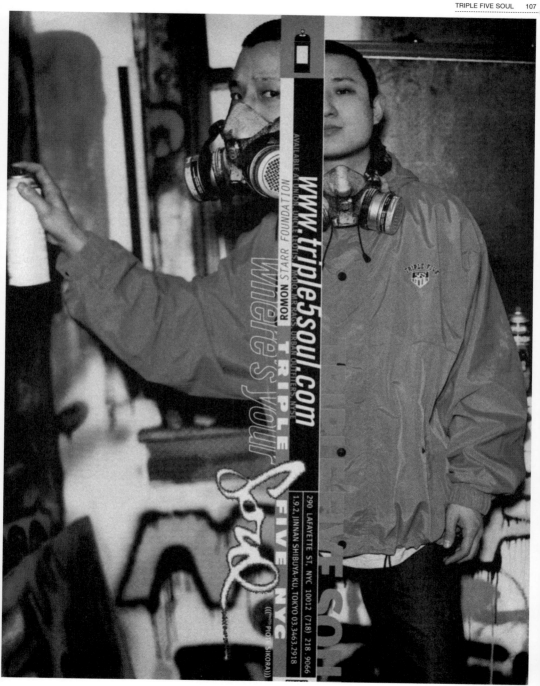

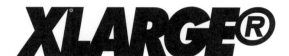

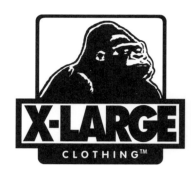

Having a Beastie Boy as one of your backers is the kind of credibility that many streetwear brands would kill for. "No Mike D, no X-Large – he is our spiritual adviser," as the brand's owner and true founder (with Adam Silverman) Eli Bonerz has graciously put it. However, X-Large, which launched in 1991 with Beastie Michael Diamond one of its shareholders, has transcended that attachment, blending its skate, hip-hop and art references to become a definitive streetwear brand. By its own definition, "true streetwear is utilitarian first and fashion-minded second. And in that sense, X-Large has always considered itself streetwear," as Rory Wilson, its long-term art director said. But X-Large is as distinct as it is functional, with the environment of the city of Los Angeles, where it is based and which is Bonerz's hometown, having played a key part in allowing it to stand out from the crowd that has followed it.

Followed it because, along with the likes of Stussy, Freshjive, Fuct and Hysteric Glamour, X-Large can count itself among those few brands that existed before the term 'streetwear' became a marketing category. Indeed, the very name 'X-Large' seems to sum up the essence and attitude of streetwear – it is a combination of Generation X, those generations born between the early 1960s and the mid-1970s and the core original streetwear consumers, and Living Large, which seems as much a prescription for a way of existing as a description of the oversized jeans that were then one of the definitive items in the streetwear wardrobe. The X-Large logo, an ape motif that, while possibly inspired by that of Ben Davis, has certainly itself been borrowed by subsequent streetwear brands, seemed to capture a spirit of wild energy and rebellion and, applied to the t-shirts and baseball caps with which the brand launched, made for iconic items popularized by, yes, Mike D, but also by other edgy but high-profile figures such as Ice Cube.

The fact that streetwear has grown up behind X-Large – plus its sheer longevity – has given it a creative scope that it has taken full advantage of, one perhaps reflective of the breadth of Bonerz's own cultural interests: before launching his career in the Los Angeles garment industry, he played in a band called Eskimo, which released a number of successful albums. The X-Large Nation website, for example (part blog, part social networking site), was launched with the simple, groundbreaking premise that its consumers should have a voice; and X-Large has inevitably been approached for many collaborations, both with the likes of

fellow streetwear leaders Fuct and collectible model designer Michael Lau, but also with corporate heavyweights such as Timberland, Reebok and Casio. "We can transform from a t-shirt to a car to a robot to a jet and then back to a t-shirt now," as X-Large business director of more than a decade, Dave Chmielewski, put it. "We couldn't do that before."

X-Large's flagship store in Vermont Street, Los Angeles, has also become as much a showcase for artistic talent as clothing. This is the store with which the whole enterprise began – as a multi-brand retail operation selling everything utilitarian, from Adidas to Puma, Carhartt to Ben Davis. "We were one of the first LA retailers specific to the music scene, the underground answer to Melrose Avenue, selling stuff that wasn't available there," Bonerz recalled. "Now our look is all over Melrose and probably on its way out. Our first big success came when we found dead stock of old 1970s and 1980s Adidas shoes. I guess they'd be called 'old-school' now, but that's not really in my lexicon. We got them for around 20 bucks a pair and sold them for 50 bucks and we just couldn't keep them in stock."

After a spell of expansion – other retailers wanting to franchise the Bonerz style of store – that gave X-Large seven stores coast to coast across the US, the company retrenched. Unable to control the ethos of the stores as it saw fit, X-Large closed all but two and focused instead not on being purveyors of other 'leftfield' brands, but on developing its own. It was, as the history of streetwear testifies, a good move.

The clean aesthetic of X-Large products and stores belies a covert sense of humour. The graphic design, top right, at first seems to be an homage to Peter Saville's design for the cover of Joy Division's "Unknown Pleasures" album – a reproduction of recorded pulses from the first discovered pulsar star. With X-Large, pulses become mountain peaks. And what's that scaling them? The outline of an ape, a neat reference to the brand's logo.

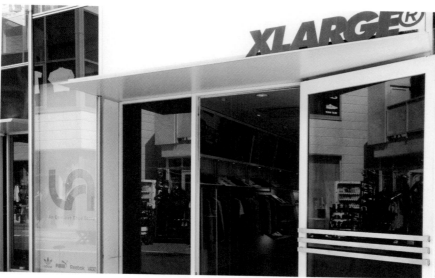
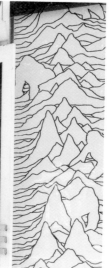

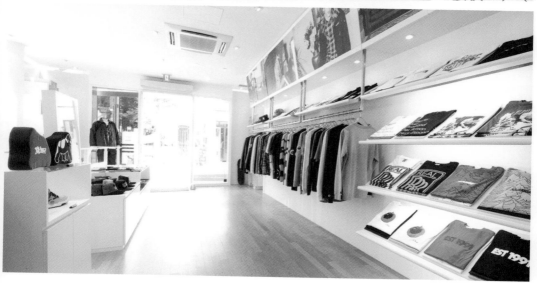

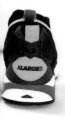
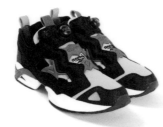
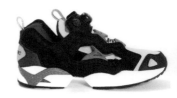

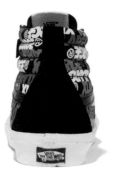

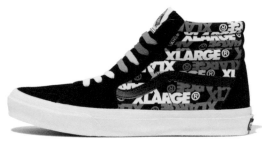

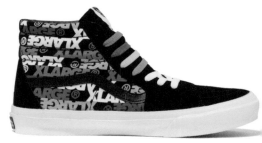

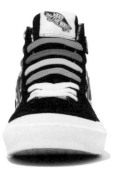

X-Large has built a reputation by making simple, utilitarian products and giving them a subtle design twist through colour or pattern, as seen in the anorak, opposite top. The same design approach has led to successful collaborations with experts in the design of functional clothing, as with the Penfield puffa jackets and gilets.

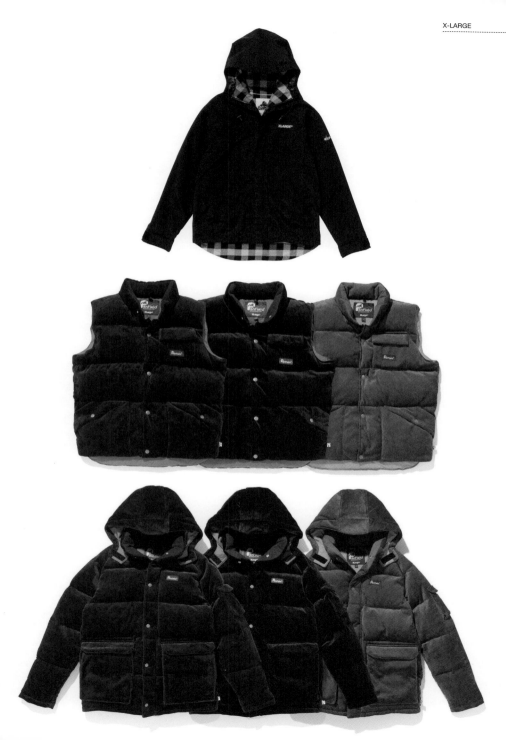

ZOO YORK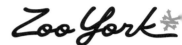

It says much about the grassroots nature of Zoo York that its name comes from a subway tunnel, built from 1971 to 1973 under New York's Central Park Zoo and a haunt of early graffiti writers. Indeed, the tunnel was so much a landmark for the budding graffiti scene that its name, the Zoo York Tunnel, or simply Zoo York, was coined by the graffiti pioneer and early rapper Ali (aka Marc André Edmonds) – with some irony. Here was a group of teenagers freely gathering in contained spaces underground, while caged animals paced above. 'Zoo York', indeed, effectively became a collective term for the city's underground movement of artists, skateboarders, B-boys and other creative sidelines.

The designs that feature on Zoo York products display a touch of nostalgia, harking back to the early days of the graffiti and skateboarding scenes and drawing a strong fan base from those with the same regard for street-culture origins. It is a nostalgia based on Zoo York's genuine heritage, rather than manufactured for marketing purposes. Although the Zoo York brand was established in 1993, its beginnings can be traced back to that early graffiti group: Zoo York co-founder Rodney Smith was one of the skateboarders and graffiti writers from the Riverside Park area of Manhattan's Upper East Side who gathered in the tunnel. In 1986 Smith and Bruno Musso created the early skateboard brand Shut Skateboards, closing that seven years later to launch Zoo York with designer Eli Morgan Gessner and businessman Adam Schatz.

Zoo York was distinctive from the outset. The products – initially just t-shirts and skateboard decks and later outerwear, denim, fleeces, footwear and accessories, for men and women – were often grittier and more rugged than those of contemporaries, blending the looks of military surplus and athletic clothing. The brand was arguably more important for its foresight rather than its clothing designs: Zoo York was key in linking action sports with street culture, blending skateboarding and graffiti with the wider worlds of BMX and surf, and later snowboard and moto-cross. It has operated professional skateboard, surf and BMX teams with a dedication usually reserved for much larger, more corporate streetwear brands. It has also maintained its connections with the graffiti world, largely through the work of the brand's later owner, Marc Ecko (aka Marc Milecofsky), the entrepreneur and founder, also in 1993, of the Ecko clothing brand.

In 2005 Ecko fought the New York City authorities all the way to Federal Court level to defend his right to hold a free outdoor graffiti art exhibition in the city, including replicas of early New York City Transit subway cars carrying work by contemporary graffiti writers. In the following year he released a hoax video of himself tagging a wing engine of Air Force One, ostensibly to draw attention to the issue of graffiti as a form of self-expression. The same year also saw him back seven graffiti artists in a lawsuit against New York City's anti-graffiti law, which banned minors from possessing spray cans and marker pens. A district judge placed a temporary injunction on the enforcement of the law, an injunction that was later upheld by the Federal appeals court.

The decision, Ecko said at the time, made a "distinction between illegal vandalism and the motif of legal graffiti as a legitimate art form that cannot be pushed aside by legislators". Such actions have, of course, added considerably to the credibility of Zoo York among streetwear fans – as they have for Ecko's other clothing lines, building on Zoo York's reputation as one of the definitive New York streetwear labels.

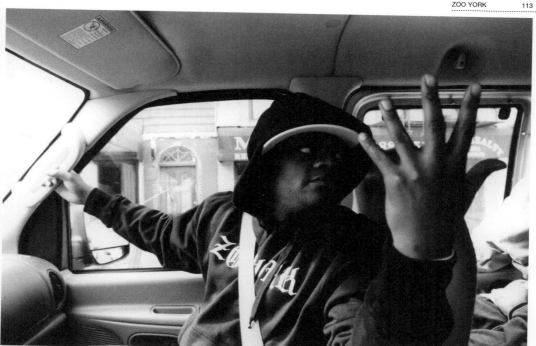

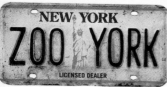

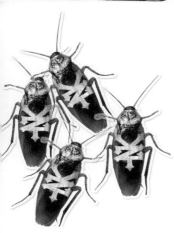

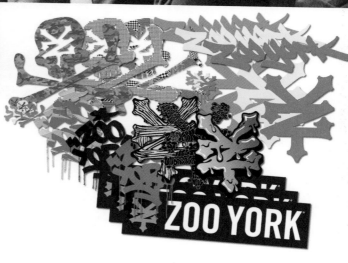

'New York, Zoo York' – the licence plate sums up the Zoo York spirit, dedicated to expressing the underground scene of New York City as a commercial enterprise. The Zoo York moniker even hints at the graphic device used by the New York Yankees baseball team, as seen on countless fans' baseball caps.

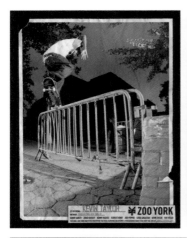

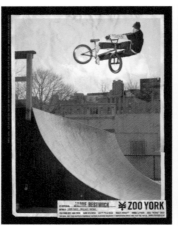

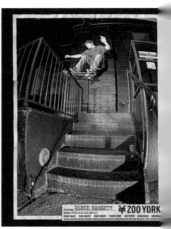

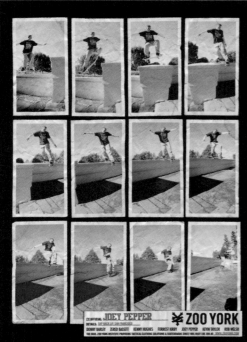

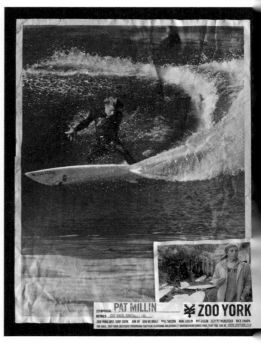

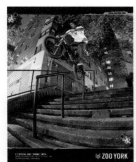
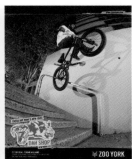

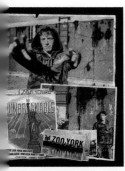
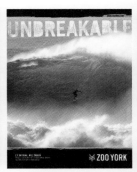

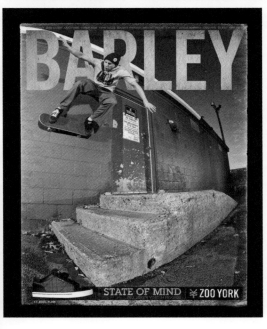

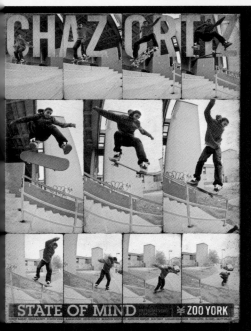

BMX, surfing and skateboarding; extreme sports with a strong street following have been central to Zoo York's pioneering (though since much copied) style. The brand has supported both professionals and local amateurs in these sports.

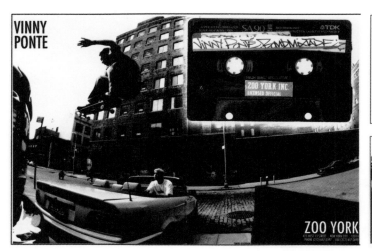

VINNY
PONTE

ZOO YORK

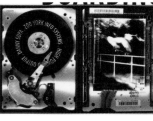

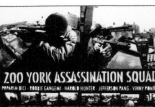

ZOO YORK ASSASSINATION SQUAD

PRPARIM BICI · ROBBIE GANGEMI · HAROLD HUNTER · JEFFERSON PANG · VINNY PONTE

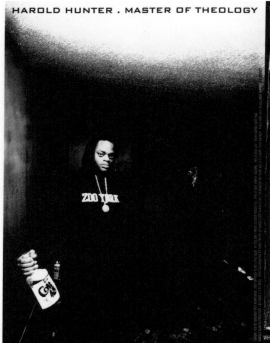

HAROLD HUNTER . MASTER OF THEOLOGY

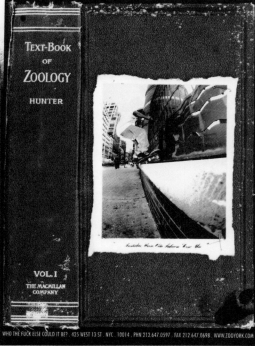

TEXT-BOOK
OF
ZOOLOGY

HUNTER

VOL. I
THE MACMILLAN
COMPANY

WHO THE FUCK ELSE COULD IT BE? . 425 WEST 13 ST . NYC . 10014 . PHN 212.647.0597 . FAX 212.647.0698 . WWW.ZOOYORK.COM

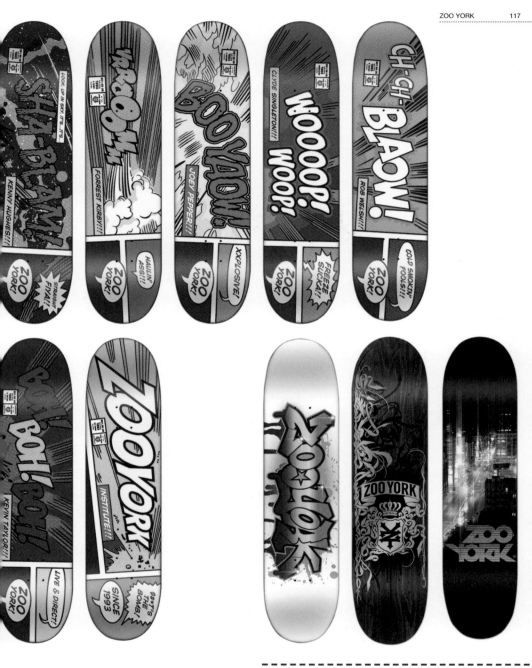

Zoo York is not alone in using skateboards as much for graphic art as to carry
wheels and skateboarders, but its connection with the sport, rather than the culture,
runs deeper than most. Zoo-York-sponsored pro skater and actor Harold Hunter,
for example, was one of the talented skaters to come out of the Brooklyn Banks
skateboard scene with Steve Cales, Dave Ortiz, Jeff Pang and the Shut Skates crew.

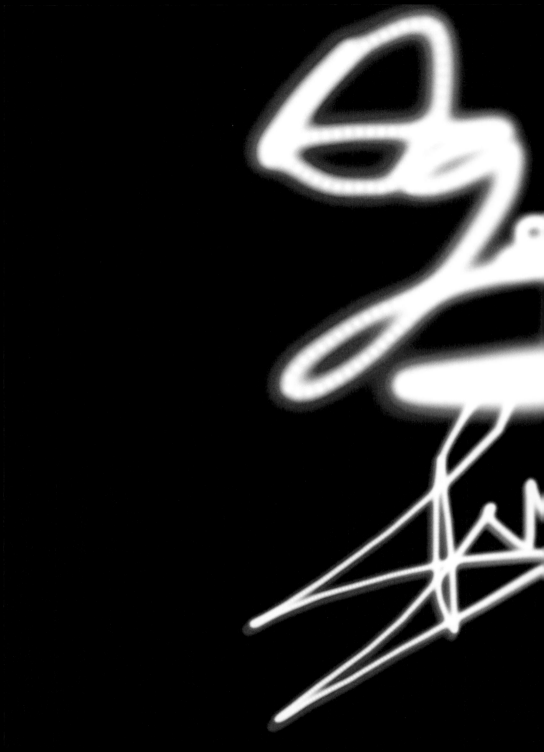

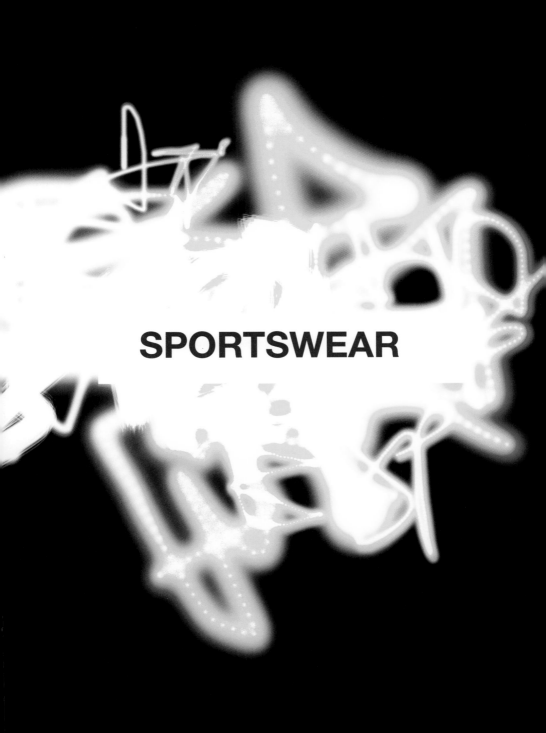

SPORTSWEAR

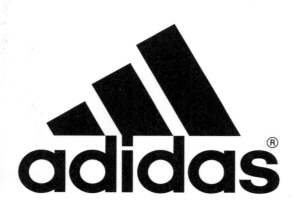

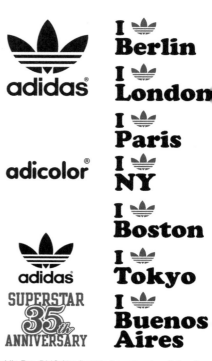

If Nike has always been reluctant to concede that its brand and product appeal are as much about fashion as they are about sport, the German company Adidas has been more than keen to admit as much, confident that interest in one does not detract from the other. In fact, its Adidas Originals business, which launched in 1991 precisely with a view to reinventing some of its retro glory, has been run, without conflict, as a separate entity from the company's sporting interests.

It is perhaps because Adidas has always been open to the idea, perhaps its European heritage, that has made the brand so central to streetwear of diverse kinds and at diverse times. This has often been subject to the availability of certain styles and the sport of choice in various places: from the 'terrace casuals' of the UK in the 1980s, with their passion for the football-oriented sneaker (or 'trainer') styles of Forest Hills or Samba (dating back to 1950), through to the basketball-oriented shoes of the New York hip-hop scene.

Hip-hop band Run-DMC, for example, were advocates of both the three-stripe tracksuit and basketball-oriented Superstars, with their distinctive shell toe, worn with the laces removed and the tongue pushed forward. They even became the subject of a song, "My Adidas" ("Now the Adidas I possess for one man is rare/myself home-boy for 50 pair/got blue and black cause I like to chill/and yellow and green when it's time to get ill"). A multi-million-dollar marketing contract followed. "We weren't trying to sell Adidas at first. I wrote a song about what was in my life," Run-DMC's Joey Simmons (aka Rev Run) noted. "We were doing what we loved and the money followed." Perhaps the appeal of Adidas sneakers comes down to the essential, almost Bauhausian simplicity of the designs – free of whistles and bells, with Adidas's three-stripe logo often the only decoration, many are streamlined styles that would not have looked out of place at any time since the 1930s.

Indeed, while Run-DMC (the first hip-hop stars to collaborate with a sportswear brand) are often cited as a turning point for the brand's acceptance into the world of streetwear, Adidas was part of street culture – or, more specifically, the music culture that underlies it – long before then. The reggae scene wore the brand, Bob Marley especially (following his passion for football), as did Jim Morrison of The Doors, Mick Jagger and Keith Richards (in Gazelle sneakers), David Bowie in his Thin White Duke period (in Stan Smiths) and Marvin Gaye (in an Adidas tracksuit) – and that was back in the days when wearing sneakers or sportswear outside the sporting arena was a genuine style statement.

Certainly more than the brand's fair share of sneaker styles have become classics. Although designed as sportswear, they made the transition to the street with ease, where they are still worn long after they become obsolete on the sports field. The Superstar, for example, was launched in 1969 as the first all-leather, low-top basketball shoe before becoming a staple of Missy Elliott, Jay-Z and Underworld (because the shoe was as much a staple of dance culture as hip-hop), the Red Hot Chili Peppers, Anthrax and Korn (because rock has also embraced the style), not to mention the characters of *Grand Theft Auto*. Hailing from the more rarefied world of tennis, the Stan Smith was designed in 1965 as the first all-leather tennis shoe and endorsed by Robert Haillet, then renamed after Smith, the US tennis player and Wimbledon champion of the late 1960s and early 1970s; it is now more of a skate shoe. Don't forget the Gazelle (1968) and suede Campus (1972) styles – the latter appearing on the cover of the Beastie Boys' "Check Your Head" album cover and one of the few sneakers ideal for the fat laces worn, as the pioneering B-boy group Rock Steady Crew once noted, to pump up the style to cartoonish proportions.

Adidas – pronounced 'addi-dass' – has a long pedigree that belies its reduction to a few sneaker styles, as classic as they may

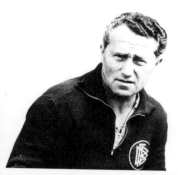

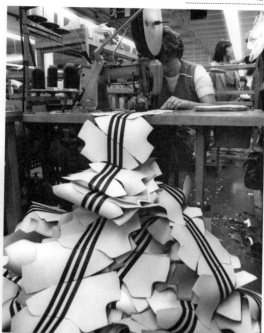

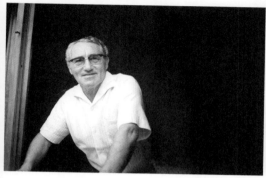

be. Adolf Dassler (known to his friends as Adi, hence the company name) started to produce his own sports shoes in his mother's kitchen in the early 1920s and was joined by his brother, Rudolf, in creating the Dassler Brothers Shoe Factory. Business was good, but the brothers' relationship was not: in 1948 Rudolf left the company to form the rival Puma. The post-war years were boom times for Adidas, especially in the realm of football. The company became the world leader in football-boot design and was manufacturer and supplier to many national football squads. Various design ventures followed, including collaborations with fashion designers Yohji Yamamoto and Stella McCartney, and the acquisition of Reebok, which put the company on a more even footing with Nike.

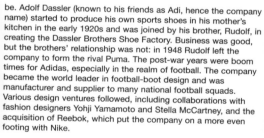

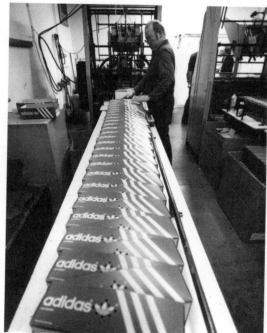

The young and the older Adolf Dassler, founder of Adidas (and from whom it takes its name), together with work inside an Adidas factory of the 1960s. The company's three-stripe graphic device, as simple as might be devised, dominates the scenes.

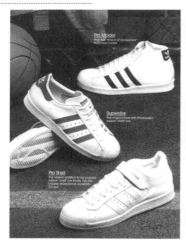

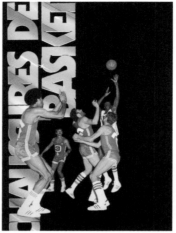

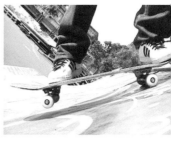

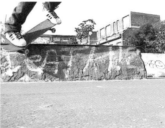

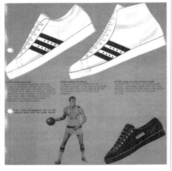

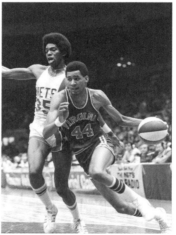

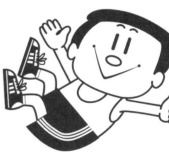

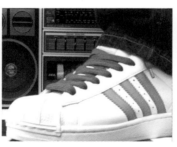

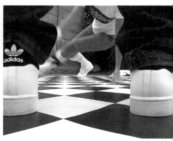

Adidas today is a brand with a foothold as much in slick fashion as in sport, counting collaborations with Yohji Yamamoto and Stella McCartney together with clinical shop-fits (opposite top). Its sporting heritage, however, has seen sneaker styles, especially those from basketball, adopted by street cultures including skate and breakdance. Opposite: sewn-on patches.

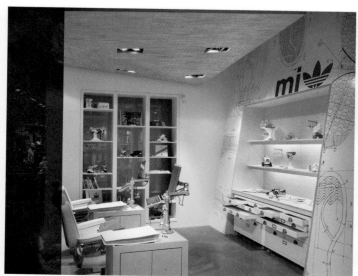
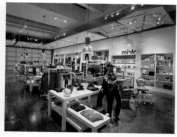
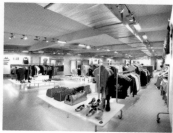

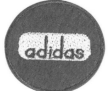
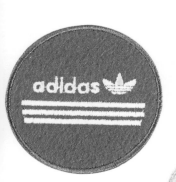
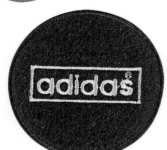

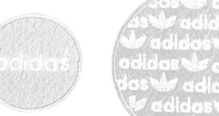

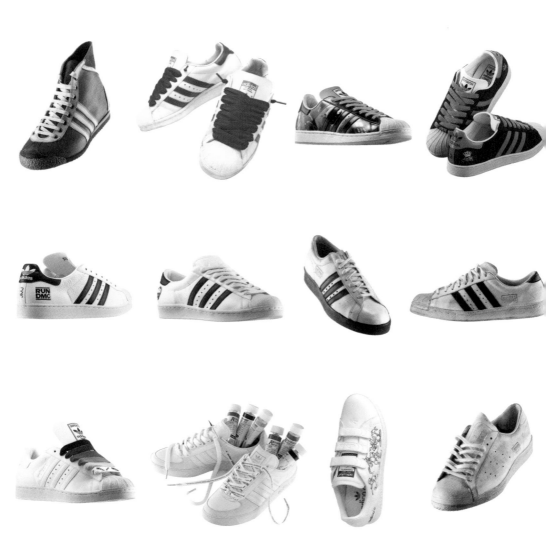

There is old-school, top left, an original Adidas basketball design from the 1960s (and potential forebear of the Gazelle), and then there is old-skool: the doyen of Adidas sneakers, the Superstar (released in 1969), more commonly known as the 'shell toe', in various incarnations, including styles produced in collaboration with Run-DMC. Other styles featured include Forest Hills (second row centre), Adicolor (1985) (bottom row centre left, complete with pens to allow the wearer to colour in the stripes) and the Velcro-strap version of the Stan Smith (mid-1990s, based on the original launched in 1968; bottom row centre right).

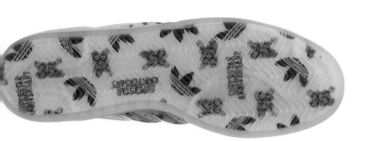
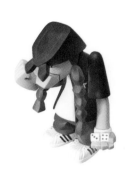

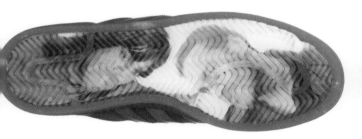
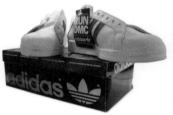

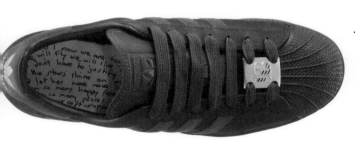
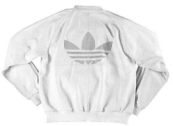

Adidas has created classic sportswear as well as sneakers, including the three-stripe/trefoil track top. Other designs include pioneering injection-moulding techniques that allow imagery to be worked into the sole, and collaborations with the likes of Missy Elliott (bottom shoe).

burton

BURTON

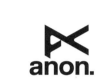

If skateboarding has been the urban sport at the heart of streetwear, then fast on its tail (via the surfboards of Stussy) is snowboarding. And that puts Jake Burton right at the forefront of street style, even though he would prefer to be out on the snow (when the snow falls heavily in Burlington, Vermont, the home of his business, everyone gets the day off to perfect their jibs, halfpipe spins, rodeo flips and cripplers). Burton – full name Jake Burton Carpenter – is the Burton of Burton Snowboards which, since 1997, has been a performance clothing label adopted as much off the piste as on it by boarders and non-boarders alike, both drawn to the functionality that is a large part of the appeal of much streetwear.

One of the sport's true pioneers, Burton had little business experience when he took his first entrepreneurial steps: he and a friend had set up a successful landscaping business with "an old station wagon, a couple of rakes and some trash bags". They spent a year assisting a large New York company that specialized in takeovers – perhaps an unlikely job for someone thinking of launching into the part rebel, part hippy world of extreme sports. Indeed, snowboarding was still an underground activity (much as skateboarding had been, and somehow carrying a similar anti-social stigma about it), when, with some inheritance money, he opened the first snowboard factory in a farmhouse in 1977. It was, in some ways, a flashback to Burton's youth, when as a 14-year-old he first surfed over the fairways of the local golf course on his Snurfer – the short, narrow proto-snowboard created in 1965 by Sherman Poppen, a man who could have become the Burton of his day had his product not, initially disastrously, been marketed to hardware rather than sports-goods stores. In fact, Burton's arrival was perhaps best summed up at the 1979 National Snurfing Championships, where he turned up with his own board, persuaded judges to create an 'open' division, and then proceeded to win it.

If the intimate link between skateboarding and streetwear lies in the fact that both grew out of small, grassroots initiatives that put a passion for the activity and the product above business interests, then Burton can certainly lay claim to almost single-handedly shaping the scene that also produced snowboarding. It was Burton, for example, who, after years of gentle pressure, successfully lobbied ski resorts to allow snowboarders access – until then, most resorts banned the sport. He also launched the US Open, the first step to recognizing snowboarding as a legitimate sport (and, since 1998, a crowd-pulling Winter Olympic event).

Burton is as keen to protect the youth culture that surrounds snowboarding as he is to perfect the research and development behind the boards and the sport itself, which only came to prominence in the 1990s, some decade and a half after he started out. "It's a lifestyle business and that means fashion is destined to be part of it. Style and expression have always been super aspects of the sport," he said. "But that doesn't mean you feel obligated to make shit that doesn't work. And we have to be careful that snowboarding doesn't become elitist, as skiing did, with all the magazines not about hardcore skiing but about which resort had the best food, or which roofrack would fit on your BMW. It ceased to be youth-driven and became class- or status-driven. Snowboarding can't fall into that trap."

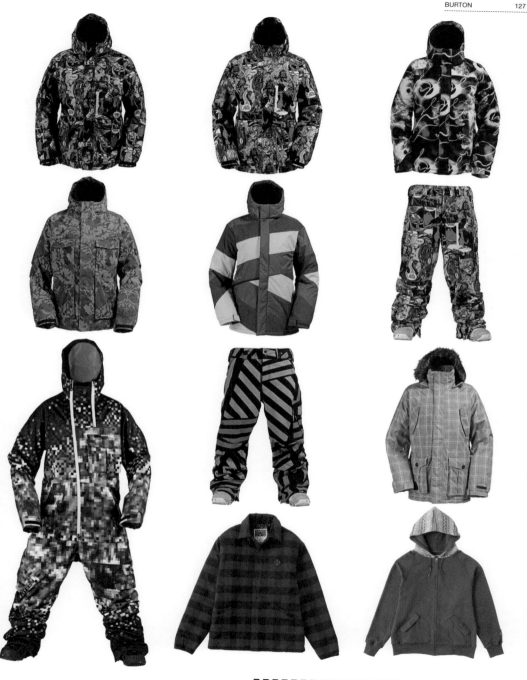

Burton's reputation for snowboarding clothing rests not only on its technical skill but the boldness of its graphic design. It would be hard to get lost in the snow in these.

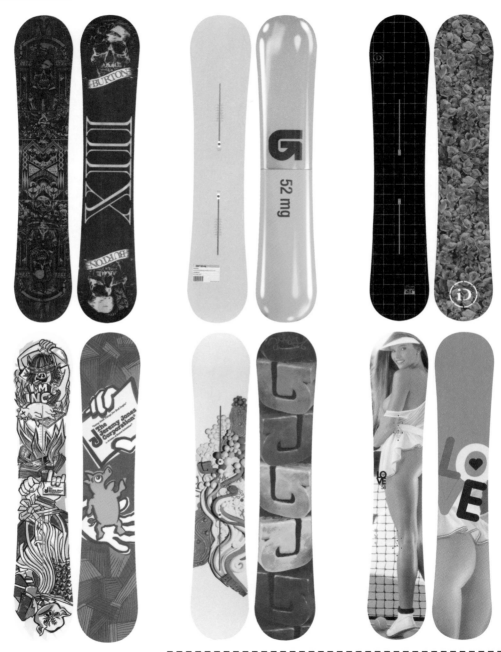

Burton began life as a maker of snowboards and, like skateboards before them, the kit has become a repository for art, from the predictable graffiti styles through to the humorous (the pill) and retro – an homage to the best-selling poster of the 1970s, 'tennis girl'.

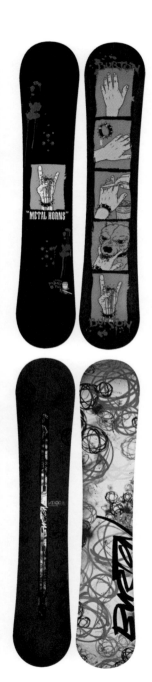

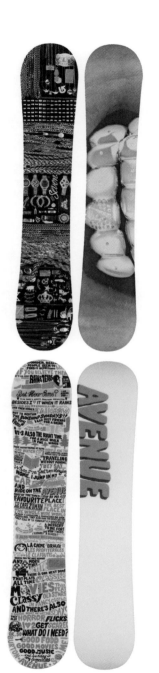

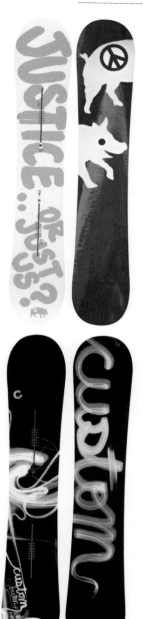

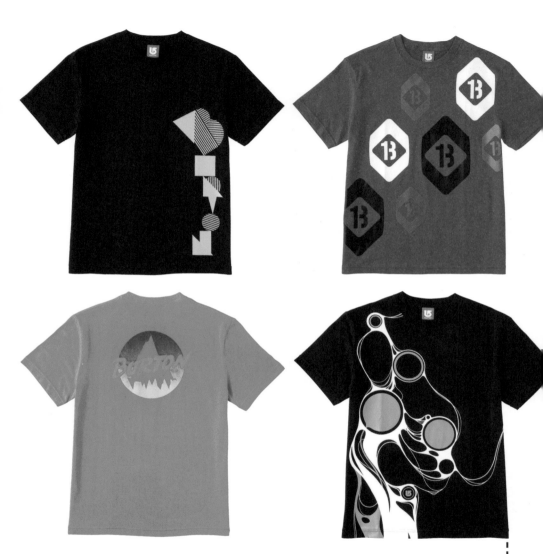

Although warm-weather clothing is not fit for
purpose for Burton's core audience, the brand has
sufficient appeal that its logo, in many forms, is
suitable fodder for t-shirts.

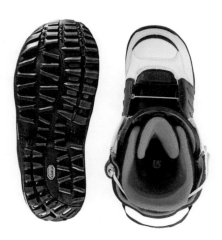

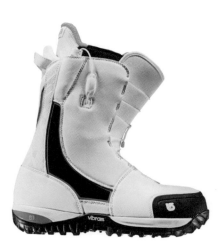

Burton's remit as a supplier to professional snowboarders means it offers a full range of high-spec equipment, including boots and, designed in collaboration with Anon, snow goggles.

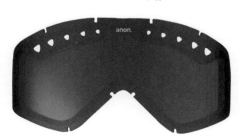

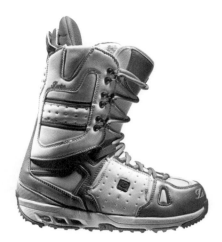

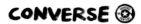

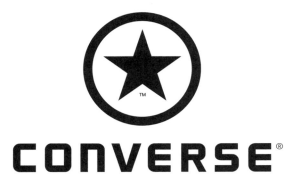

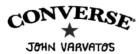

Before Nike's Jordan or Puma's Clyde came a basketball shoe that defined the very idea of footwear designed for specialist, athletic purposes but worn more in the urban environment. In this respect, Marquis Mills Converse was ahead of the game. The manager of a footwear company, in 1908 he decided to go it alone and launch his own business – the Converse Rubber Shoe Company, based in Malden, Massachusetts. Converse quickly established a strong reputation making gents' rubber-soled shoes, breaking into the tennis-shoe market in 1915 and launching the Converse All Star basketball shoe two years later. It was a groundbreaking shoe.

In other ways, however, Marquis Converse may have missed the boat. The story goes that, in 1921, an established basketball player by the name of Charles, or 'Chuck', Taylor walked into Converse's Chicago offices looking for a job. Converse didn't sign him up as the new face of their product. These, after all, were the days before celebrity ruled the world. Rather, the company hired Taylor as a salesman, only thinking to add his name to the shoe during the 1930s, making it the first ever signature basketball shoe (though not one worn by an active player). The period also saw Converse launch another sneaker to find retro appeal decades later: the Jack Purcell court shoe, designed by the badminton champ of the same name in 1935.

That Taylor got to put his name to an iconic product, however, was a reward for work to come: he suggested the patch to protect the ankle, ensured that Chuck Taylors were the official PT (physical training) shoe of the US Army during the Second World War and launched the first Converse Basketball Clinic – this was not only

a way of improving the basketball skills of college kids across the US, but also a means of encouraging coaches and local sporting-goods stores to make a switch to Converse boots. By 1949 he had also turned them into the official footwear for every player in the National Basketball League (the forerunner of the National Basketball Association).

Indeed, Taylor was a salesman and frontman for the basketball shoe for some 48 years, until his death in 1969. More importantly, he also oversaw the All Star boot's becoming part of American folklore, such that a pair of the simple canvas boots – which were only available in black until 1947, when an all-white version was introduced – became as much part of the teenage (though the term had yet to be invented) and collegiate uniform as denim and checked flannel shirts, not to mention a choice of the era's rockabilly subculture (then and now, in fact). This was due largely to some clever marketing: each year the company produced the *Converse Yearbook*, which celebrated the highlights of the basketball year, including high-school athletics, and came complete with illustrations by Charles Kerins, whose work, along with that of Norman Rockwell, created the archetypal imagery of the 1950s American Dream.

Add it all up and it meant that by the 1960s Converse dominated the athletics footwear market. In 1966 the company even decided to introduce seven colour options for the boot. The time at the top, however, was short-lived, as other athletics footwear companies launched through the 1970s and Converse failed to innovate. The Converse high-top was eclipsed by the

athlete Chuck Taylor lent his name to of the biggest-selling sneaker styles of all time, emblazoned with the star logo at the heel and barely changed since it was launched in the 1930s.

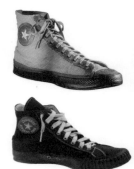

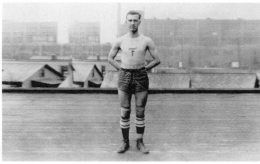

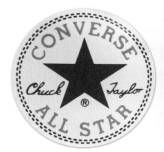

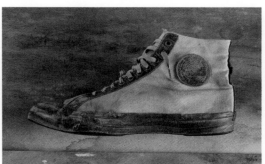

kes of Nike's Air Force 1 and the Adidas Superstar. Even the unch in 1974 of the One Star sneaker, which became a kateboard staple, was not enough.

That, however, has never stopped Chuck Taylor from retaining e affection of many fans – who, by turns, have referred to them s 'Chuckies', 'Connies' and 'Cons' – or being well-worn by key, pically music-led, subcultures from the late 1970s onwards, cluding American punk rock, grunge, G-funk, the bass-heavy ariety of American West Coast rap/hip-hop and, at the turn of e 21st century, the goth-esque style of hardcore punk/emo, l of which has driven a Converse revival, keeping Chuck Taylor otwear, in particular, part of streetwear. While the canvas onstruction has always made them ready for customization, e appeal of Chucks was only likely to increase following the urchase of Converse by Nike in 2003. By then, however, they ould long ago have comfortably claimed to be the best-selling thletics shoe of all time.

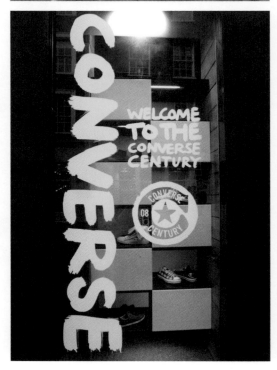

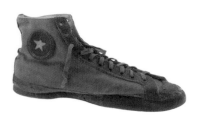

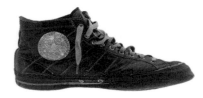

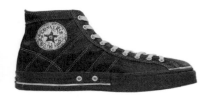

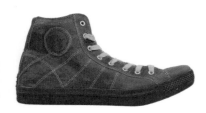

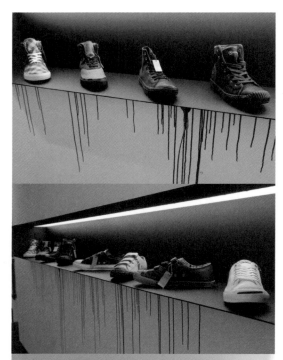

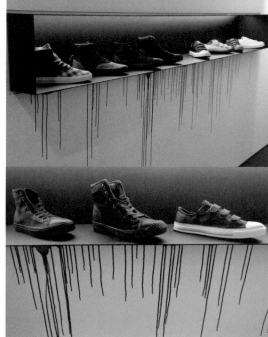

Four styles of the original Converse Chuck Taylor model, made with leather uppers before the famous canvas version was introduced, and a long way from the high-tech basketball boots designed for today's players.

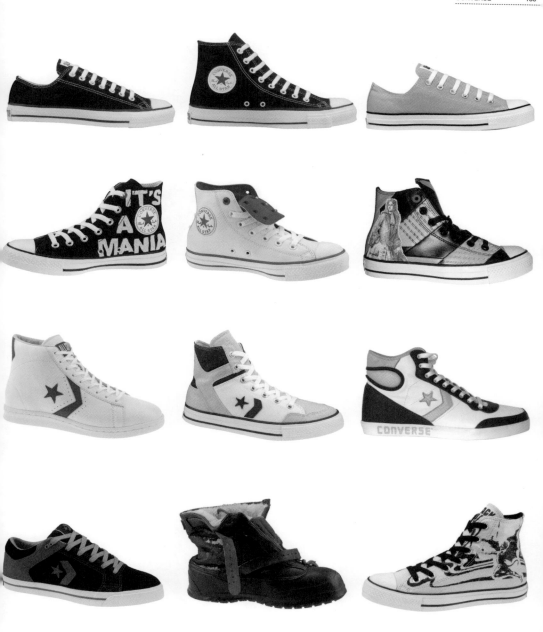

While Converse has created more technical basketball shoes, such as the One Star line (third row: Pro Leather, Poorman and Fastbreak), and specialist pieces such as the pilot's boot made during the Second World War, bottom row centre, its reputation is built on the Chuck Taylor. This comes in two basic models, low- and high-top, the upper proving a literal blank canvas not just for graphic artists, but also the owners – biro has long been a means of personalization. Converse's collaboration with (PRODUCT) RED has also led to new styles.

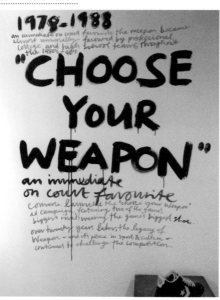

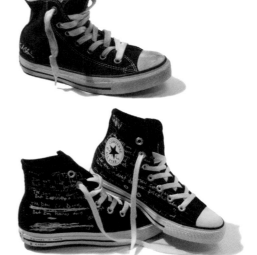

This in-store advertisement tells the story of The Weapon, the basketball boot of choice among college and professional players during the late 1970s. The company's promotional campaign pitched the best players in opposition, with both wearing the sleek and timeless shoe.

Aside from Elvis Presley, who wore Jack Purcells, perhaps Converse's most famous fan was Nirvana's Kurt Cobain, who helped make Chuck Taylors part of the 1990s grunge wardrobe. Such was his influence that Converse issued a pair scrawled with his lyrics.

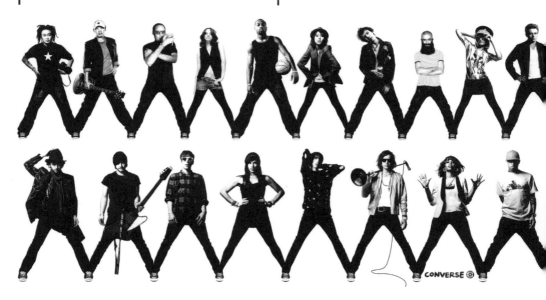

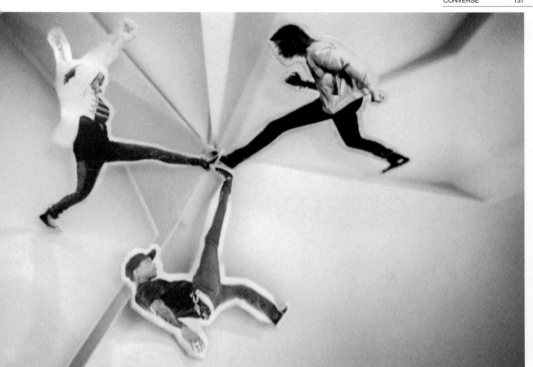

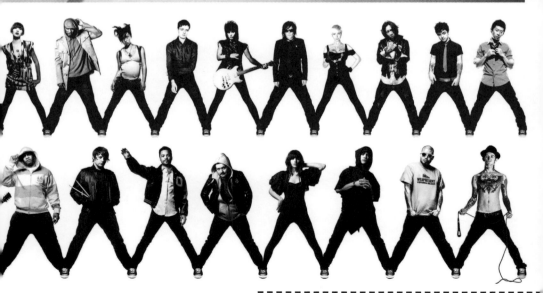

In 2008, Converse celebrated their centennial with the Connectivity campaign, above. The advertising visually connects past and present Converse icons, brought together by the Chuck Taylor. The paper-chain-style pictures here make a point of the shoe's popularity among musicians, including Green Day's frontman Billie Joe Armstrong.

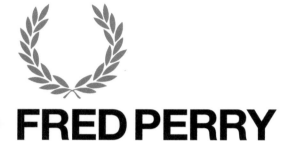

FRED PERRY

It was not the best marketing idea in the world. When British tennis ace and three times Wimbledon champion Fred Perry wanted to launch a sportswear line under his own name, his first idea for a logo was a pipe. As a keen pipe-smoker (and product of the times) he failed to see the irony in what could be interpreted as the implement of a cancer-inducing habit being used for clothing in which vigorous activity was intended. It was Perry's Austrian business partner (and one-time footballer), Tibby Wegner, who scotched the idea and suggested the wreath embroidered on Perry's Davis Cup sweater.

Not all of Perry's marketing ideas had been off-kilter, however. On turning pro, he toured the US, made a small fortune from exhibition matches, bought the Beverly Hills Tennis Club and made profits soar by installing a bevy of beauties around the pool. He taught tennis to the Hollywood greats but in the 1940s broke his wrist and needed a new career. Luck had it that Wegner had approached Perry for endorsement of an innovative product he had designed for players – the first sweatband made out of a heavy towelling. But it grew heavier the wetter it got – not, in other words, ideal for tennis players. Perry suggested changes to the design, Wegner found a more effective fabric and, with the new sweatband, the Fred Perry brand was born.

Wegner's next suggestion was that they manufacture a white cotton piqué polo shirt to compete with Lacoste, the French brand that had originated it. The first Fred Perry polo came out in 1952 and was destined to become iconic. Perry himself (who, cannily, always wore one of his shirts while commentating for the BBC) may not have suspected that it would become a look off-court, worn big and baggy as a key component for streetwear, especially in the UK, and especially among 'Perry boys', the working-class lads who were a long way from the 'polo' shirt and lifestyle imagined by Ralph Lauren. Perry, at least, had also been a real working-class lad made good.

Indeed, despite being worn by the great and good (including Queen Elizabeth's mother and John F. Kennedy – the only man the Fred Perry company granted the accolade of having three initials, rather than two, sewn onto his personalized shirt), 'a Perry', as the shirt came to be affectionately known, has had greater impact on street culture, arguably making the transition from sport to street long before tracksuits or trainers. The Perry was an integral part of Mod style, worn under slimline tailoring; and that of skinheads, worn with Doc Marten boots, braces and rolled Levi's – both the original skinheads, who took their inspiration from the reggae fans who first wore the shirt in black dance clubs, and the far-right variety who came to sully the image of their (apolitical) sartorial forebears. It was part of the style of soul boys and the band The Casuals in the 1980s, when it was put under a V-neck sweater; and it was also worn by British skaters. Few items of clothing can claim to have a place in so many diverse youth subcultures as a statement of clan membership.

Latterly, the Perry has been inspiring for the high-fashion designers Jil Sander and Comme des Garçons, but it has never been dropped by its more working-class leanings (however faux they may be), nor lost its connection with music. The Specials and Paul Weller, but also Blur and Mike Skinner, better known as rapper The Streets, carried Perry-wearing through 'new rave' and into the new British indie scene of the mid-2000s.

Fred Perry has transcended its sporting roots, but it will always have an attachment to tennis, through its tennis star founder Fred Perry (in action centre row) or through more recent fashion-aware tennis collections.

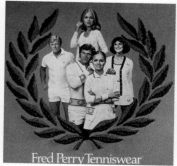

Fred Perry Tenniswear

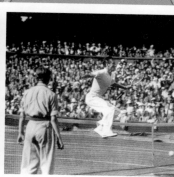

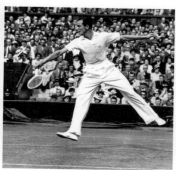

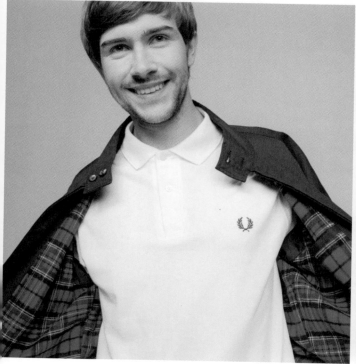

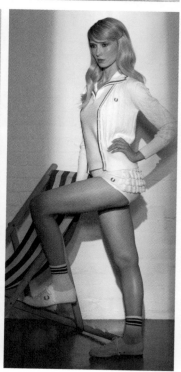

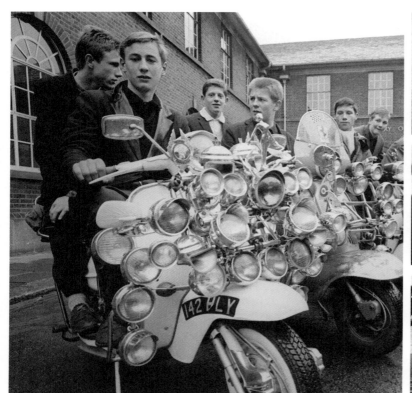

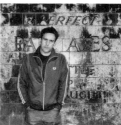

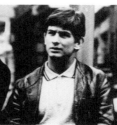

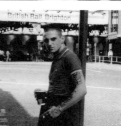

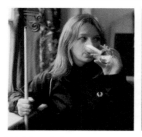

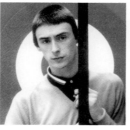

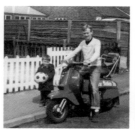

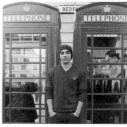

Although also worn by the Skinhead style movement of the 1970s and later by Casuals during the 1980s, it was the Mod scene that drove Fred Perry's transition from sports to style star. A 'Perry' was the shirt of choice for the original Mods, top, and has been for Mod acolyte and hero Paul Weller (bottom row second from left).

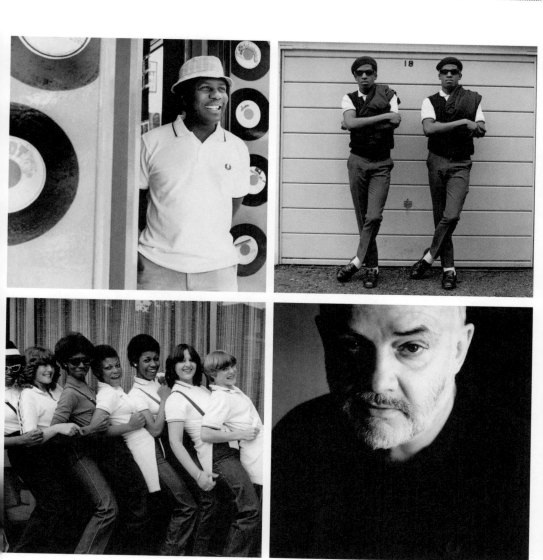

Fred Perry won a dedicated following including DJ Norman Jay (top left), John Peel (bottom right) and The Specials' Terry Hall (opposite top right).

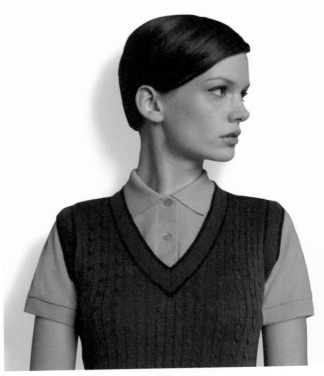

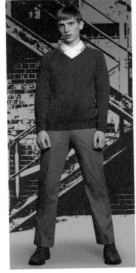

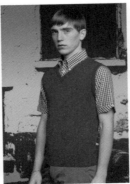

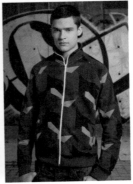

Fred Perry has established itself as a fashion brand with a full collection, but its polo shirt remains its bedrock. With it come hints of Mod, with even contemporary advertising campaigns nodding to the sartorial exactitude of the 1960s movement.

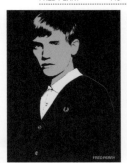

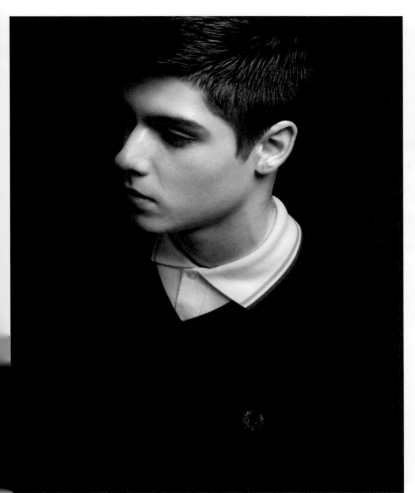

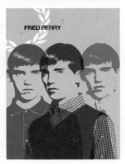

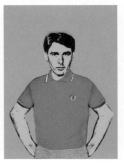

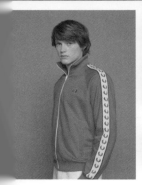

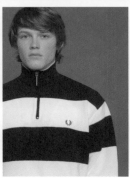

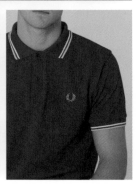

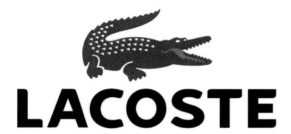

LACOSTE

It may not have the might of a Nike, but this smaller French company can take the title of the world's first sportswear brand. Indeed, back when Phil Knight, Nike's founder, was yet to do anything, French tennis ace René Lacoste was setting up a company with a product and marketing strategy so groundbreaking it would come to overshadow his achievements on the court. And that's as winner of seven Grand Slam singles titles.

Yes, his company would create the first steel tennis racquet and the first shock dampener. But it would also pioneer an idea that would prove rather popular in later decades: putting a brand logo on the outside of a garment. The logo was, of course, the alligator, a version of the badge Lacoste had been wearing on his blazer since 1927 in honour of the nickname he was accorded after playing for a set of alligator cases in a bet with the captain of the French Davis Cup team. It is, by any account, a strange logo – a seemingly smiling, cuddly yet killer reptile, drawn by artist Robert George. But in effectively inventing what marketing types call 'exterior branding', it set a benchmark for all the streetwear brands to follow. Certainly, with so much streetwear generic in terms of product design (fundamentally founded on menswear basics), branding has been crucial to its success.

But the logo – much counterfeited – was not the only revolutionary sartorial touch or contribution to casual dressing: what the logo was on would give rise to an icon for streetwear and beyond. If, pre-Lacoste, tennis was played in starched, full-sleeved shirts, young René wore what he called a polo shirt in lightweight, breathable cotton known as 'jersey petit piqué'. After joining forces with knitwear manufacturing entrepreneur André Gillier in 1933, the polo shirt went into production, initially available only in white. The polo shirt, in Lacoste's case known as the '12-12', has subsequently become a streetwear icon, a dressy but still casual alternative to the t-shirt, produced in one version or another by most streetwear brands and those that have become part of streetwear style (most notably, Ralph Lauren Polo). It's one that appeals to diverse street cultures internationally.

After all, the polo shirt, with its soft ribbed collar, often worn turned up, and its 'tennis tail' – the shirt is longer at the back so that it remains tucked in while serving – is seen on the backs of Euro hip-hop kids in the *banlieues*, or suburbs, of Paris, via the baggy rave scene of 1990s Manchester, and became a staple for West Coast skaters as much as for the preppy set of Long Island New York. It reveals streetwear's history of appropriating styles from across the social spectrum, from the upper crust as much as the industrial worker, and taking them to urban streets. No wonder Lacoste sells many hundreds of millions of dollars' worth of the 12-12 every year. The polo shirt remains a streetwear staple – in and out of favour, according to the style's vacillations between the bold, graphic and colourful, and the more clean-lined, sophisticated and sober, and still considered the perfect place for branding, as Ralph Lauren demonstrated in the late 2000s by producing a style with an outsized, embroidered logo.

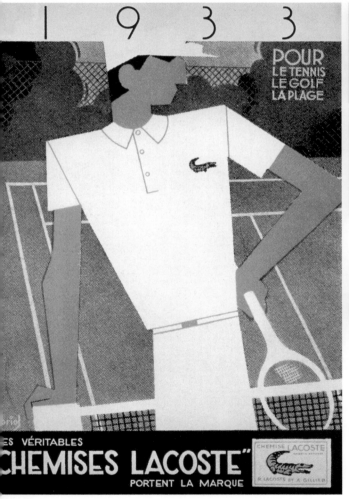

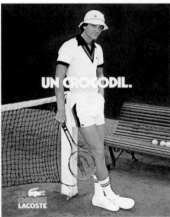

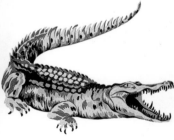

The alligator logo has become one of the most widely counterfeited in fashion, a backhanded compliment to the brand's power – especially since, hailing from tennis of the 1920s, its reputation is essentially built on one item, the cotton piqué polo shirt that it pioneered.

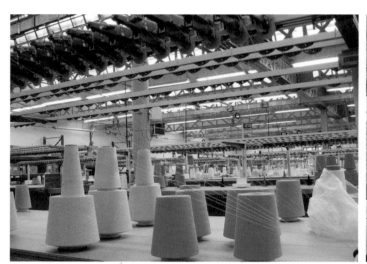

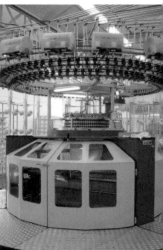

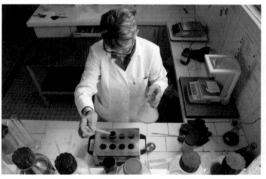

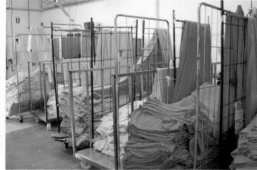

Although Lacoste has put its famed badge to other styles of clothing now, including sneakers and dressier clothes, its basic, plain, two-button 12-12 polo shirt remains its best-seller. Enormous effort is put into colour design and high-tech dyeing.

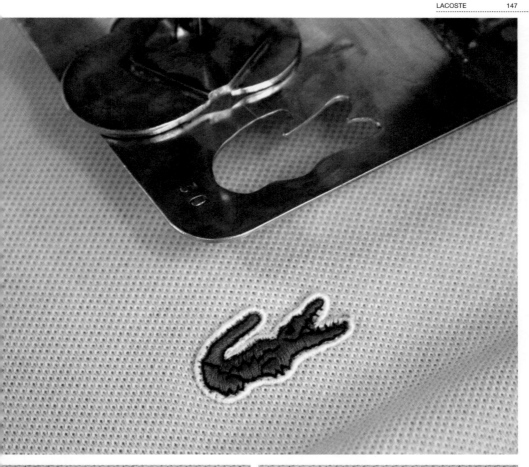

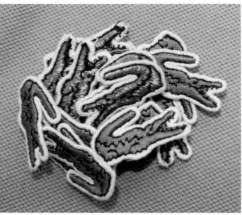

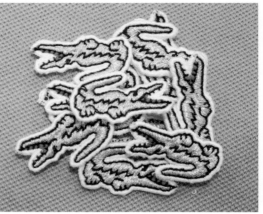

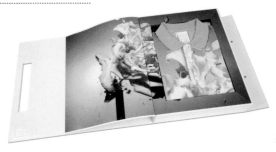
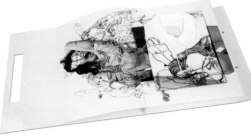

Lacoste has built a more modern image through collaborations with creatives outside the fashion industry. Special-edition polo shirts to celebrate Lacoste's 75th anniversary were designed by photographers Nick Knight, Phil Poynter, Ines van Lamsweerde, Vinoodh Matadin and Peter Lindbergh, designer Karl Lagerfeld, film director Pedro Almodóvar, illustrator Richard Phillips and REM frontman Michael Stipe, among others.

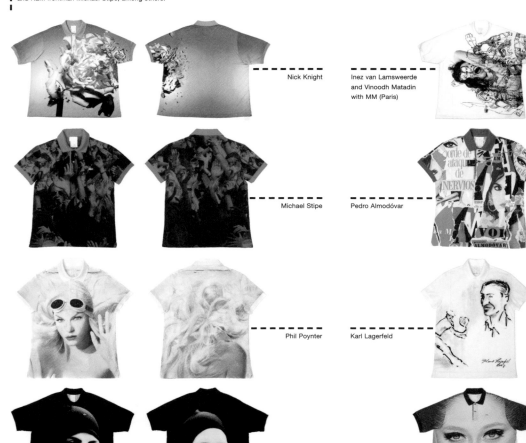

Nick Knight

Inez van Lamsweerde and Vinoodh Matadin with MM (Paris)

Michael Stipe

Pedro Almodóvar

Phil Poynter

Karl Lagerfeld

Peter Lindbergh

Richard Phillips

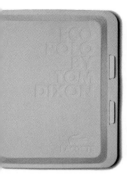

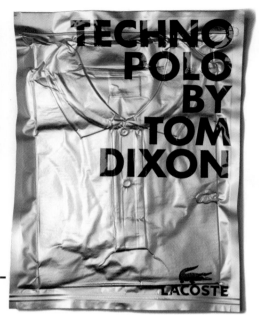

TECHNO POLO BY TOM DIXON

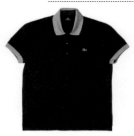

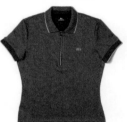

2006, British product designer Tom ...on worked on the first Lacoste ...iday Collector series – aiming to ...allenge traditional production methods ...ll processes – to produce two styles ...polo, Eco and Techno.

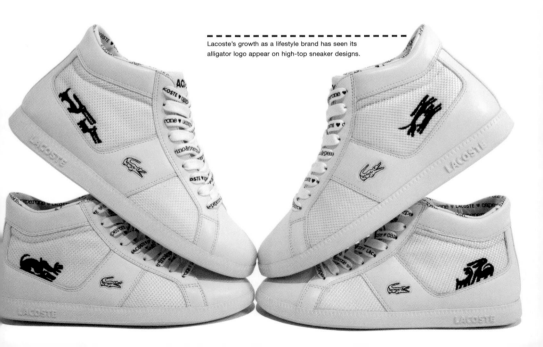

Lacoste's growth as a lifestyle brand has seen its alligator logo appear on high-top sneaker designs.

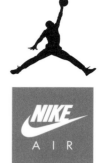

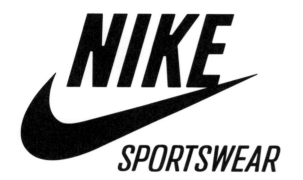

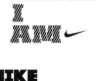

Nike may be one of the world's biggest sportswear brands, but what its monolithic corporate size loses in terms of grassroots intimacy, of the kind the streetwear world typically appreciates, it makes up for with sheer design potency. While its sweats and specialist clothing have their followers, it is Nike's sneakers that have made the brand a footwear benchmark in streetwear terms. Certainly, by launching a dialogue between designers, brand and star athletes, Nike turned utilitarian shoes into status items and invented modern sports marketing into the bargain.

Indeed, Nike has more than its fair share of sneaker icons in its portfolio: the Dunk, for example, became the default street sneaker of choice. Originally introduced in the US in 1985 as a basketball shoe, the Dunk came in 12 colours, each unique to the college team it represented – but colour not only tapped into the fashion of the decade, it gave another avenue for more personal expression. Meanwhile, Nike's close association with higher education – at one time more than 60 of the US's leading colleges were supplied with Nikes – gave the shoe unparalleled youth recognition. But it was the style's broad base and low profile that made it a hit with skateboarders as much as basketballers, such that the company even launched a dedicated skateboard version, the puffy-tongued Nike SB Dunk.

Nike's selection of what, more in retrospect than at the time, has become a pantheon of sneaker styles capable of transcending the mother brand, is long: to name just a few, the Air Carnivore

(originally set to be named the Air-Odactyl), the Air Diamond Turfs (widely considered the prototype 'cross-training' shoe), the Air Stab, the minimalistic Air Loom, and the fantastically titled Air Conditioner. Each has its own fan base and folklore.

Similarly, any sneaker fiend will know, for example, that the Air Force 1 basketball shoe – one of the most collectible sneakers ever, with box-fresh original examples (rather than more recent reissues, such as that of the Dunk in 1998) changing hands for thousands of dollars – was first designed by Bruce Kilgore in the late 1970s and was one of the first styles to cross over from sport to street, to be worn by the likes of rappers Snoop Dogg and Jay-Z. Likewise, the Air Max 90 was one of a classic series of sneakers launched in 1987, designed by Tinker Hatfield, who is little short of being a god to the legions of sneaker fanatics. It went on to become a streetwear staple.

The company has always been keen to stress its impressive technological credentials – Hatfield was the first sneaker designer to use, for example, neoprene, while even Nike founder Bill Bowerman is said to have created the Nike Waffle sole by pouring modelling clay into a waffle iron. But these developments have often resulted in stylistic leaps too: Hatfield's Air gaseous cushioning system, like Paris's Pompidou Centre before it, or the iMac after, put the insides on show. Such has been the breadth of Nike's ability to shoe the world that it is little exaggeration when Hatfield says: "I've been all around the world on trips and there

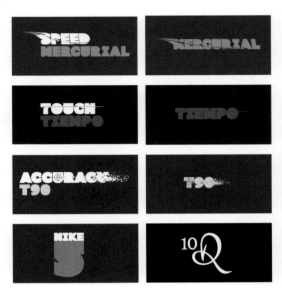

was no place where I didn't see something I designed. Maybe that's testament to brand power. But I don't know how many designers could have had that kind of experience. I could never have predicted how sneakers could influence popular culture or be a means of self-expression. To me they've always just been about adding the romance of colour and form to problem-solving. But a large proportion of our products are purchased for fashion. We know that. You buy a Porsche because it looks beautiful but you also know that thing will get-up-and-go, even if you never drive it that way. That's part of the cachet of sports shoes: the fashion is enhanced by the fact they actually do something. It's about practical issues, with pizzazz."

Pizzazz or practicality, Hatfield also made what is perhaps the single greatest contribution to sneaker culture: he has designed 20 of the Jordan line sneakers (Peter Moore designed the very first), improved on with the Dunk but still the Holy Grail of street footwear. The Jordan, affectionately known as 'Js' or 'MJs', was not only a massive marketing success for Nike (a single ad campaign for the first shoe in streetwear-hungry Japan elevated Nike to the second-most-recognized US brand after Coca-Cola), it created a cult. And not just for Jordan, who signed a deal giving him five per cent of the wholesale price of every pair sold, but on the street.

As a Nike ad put it, after the National Basketball Association tried to ban Jordan from wearing non-regulation, coloured footwear: "On October 15th, Nike created a revolutionary new basketball shoe. On October 18th, the NBA threw them out of the game. Fortunately, the NBA can't stop you wearing them." And wear them they did. It was a cult that just kept growing: almost a decade on, in 1993, Jordan played for the Chicago Bulls wearing a pair of Hatfield's black-and-white Jordan shoes, and a fuzzy photo was printed in the regional paper. Within an hour of the paper being published, 400 people called the local Niketown store to order them.

Variations on one of the world's most famous logos, the Nike swoosh or tick, created by a graphic designer friend of Nike founder Phil Knight for a one-off payment of just a few dollars.

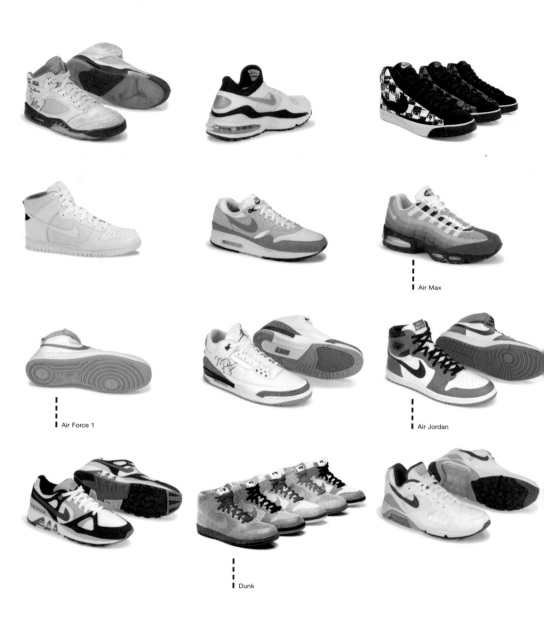

Air Max

Air Force 1

Air Jordan

Dunk

Nike's sneakers inspire fanatical collectors, with early styles, such as the Air Jordan, Air Max, Air Force 1 and Dunk inspiring particular devotion. Other styles have included the Air Presto, Air Safari and Cortez. All have their origins in the first commercial Nike sneaker, the Waffle.

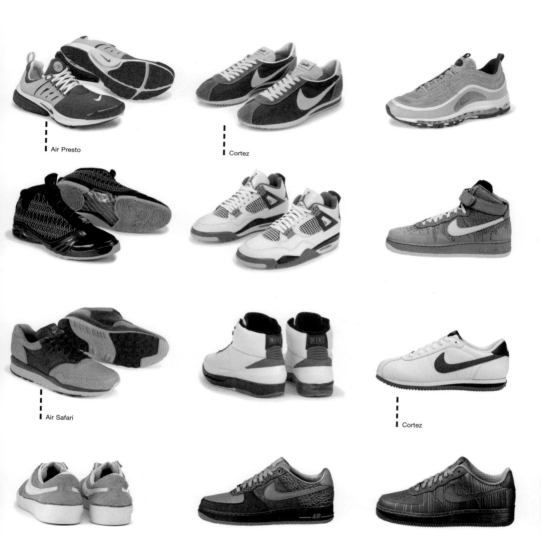

Air Presto

Cortez

Air Safari

Cortez

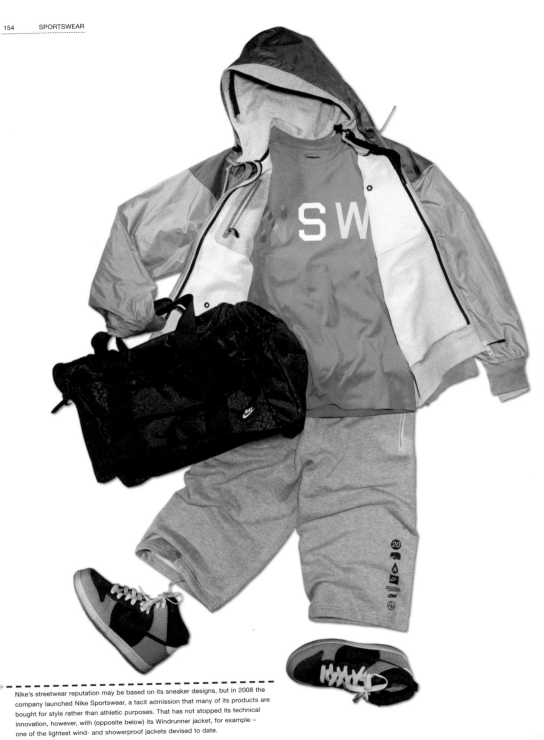

Nike's streetwear reputation may be based on its sneaker designs, but in 2008 the company launched Nike Sportswear, a tacit admission that many of its products are bought for style rather than athletic purposes. That has not stopped its technical innovation, however, with (opposite below) its Windrunner jacket, for example – one of the lightest wind- and showerproof jackets devised to date.

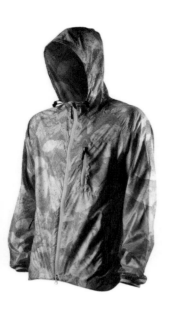

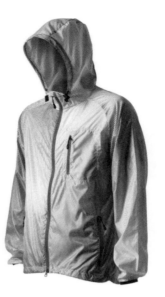

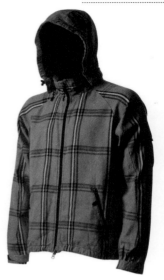

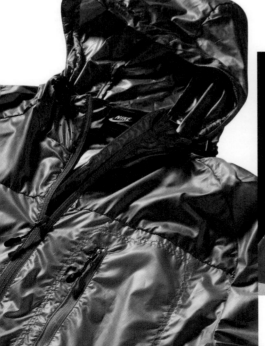

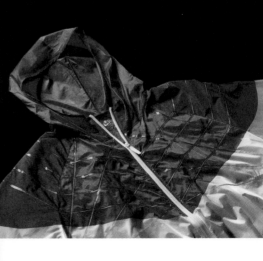

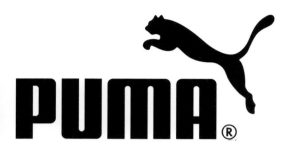

When, in 1924, brothers Rudolf and Adolf Dassler founded the Dassler Brothers Shoe Factory in Herzogenaurach, Germany, it was ostensibly to create track shoes for professionals – Jesse Owens wore their shoes to win four gold medals at the 1936 Olympic Games. By 1948, the duo had split – Adolf went off to establish Adidas – and Puma was born, turning its attention to football boots, creating the first pair with screw-in studs and beginning a long-standing relationship with the sport. All of which makes for a highly technical tradition that might not best serve the interests of style.

And yet Puma has had many hits in the world of sneaker appreciation: the Roma, the premium cowhide sneakers launched in white and royal blue to celebrate the 1968 Azzurri European Champion winners, Italy; the TX-3 running shoe of 1985; the following year's Sky II basketball shoe, with its belt-and-braces laces and Velcro fastening system for a perfect fit; even 1991's Disc, which did away with laces altogether and introduced a turning mechanism that tightened the shoe around the foot – and which never did quite work properly.

Unusually, even tennis furnished street style with two sneaker classics, notably the G Vilas, the 1977 signature shoe of the Argentine tennis ace Guillermo Vilas, with its characteristic perforated toe, and the Boris Becker Ace, launched in 1980, the signature shoe of the player who went on to be the youngest man to win Wimbledon (in 1985).

But perhaps more than any other Puma shoe, the one held in greatest affection is the Clyde, an update of Puma Suedes, launched in 1973 and worn and endorsed by New York Knicks basketball star Walt 'Clyde' Frazier (named Clyde for his Bonnie and Clyde period taste in clothing – a wide-brimmed fedora, mink coat and sneakers being just one of his looks). The style, arguably the first ever signature shoe, would come to be better, albeit unofficially, known internationally as Puma States because of the numbers imported into Europe from the US – it was a stripped-down suede sneaker seemingly available in every colour, creating in the process a street style hunt for matching wide laces, which were then typically worn flat, loose and pristine. "It wasn't just a basketball shoe," as Frazier recalled. "You could style this shoe, that's why I endorsed it – it had to look cool to me. And whatever I had on the court, you could bet that the next day the kids would be out wearing that type of shoe."

Indeed, Clydes were not only one of the first sneakers to cross from sports to leisure wear (worn colour-matched with your socks), but would become an essential component of the B-boy/breakdance uniform – DJ Cash Money kept his cleaner longer by buying dark-coloured pairs, but then required a constant supply of new white socks as the dye from the sneaker marked them, while Grandmaster Melle Mel of the Furious Five has noted that scuffing your Clydes was a good indicator that you hadn't perfected a breakdance move.

Clydes were also simple and light – ideal for evading the authorities when caught tagging trains, making them the choice of 1970s NYC graffiti legends such as Stay High 149. "For me the Clyde represents when sneakers got fly," as hip-hop icon Fab Five Freddie has put it. "Suddenly they really made you stand out from the crowd. And [in suede] they were more of a challenge to keep clean so you had to have multiple pairs."

Multiple pairs also had to be made to meet demand: as hip-hop borrowed from punk and punk sub-genres borrowed from hip-hop, the Clyde style crossed back and forth across what at first may seem opposing cliques. Skateboarders, meanwhile, would seek out a harder-wearing version in the guise of Puma Basket, the Clyde re-imagined in leather. Casual terrace and acid jazz fashion would again pick up on the Clyde during the early 1980s.

Frazier himself, fittingly, had always been a proto-sneakerhead, before the birth of the streetwear market. "When I was 10 or 11, my sneakers were the hottest things in my wardrobe," he said. "I used to wash them with soap and brush them every night so they would be bright and dry by morning. I remember being very excited about how I laced them up. I was full of pride when I used to wear my sneakers. I dug looking down and catching myself walking in them."

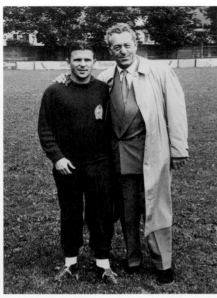

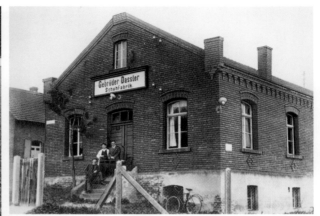

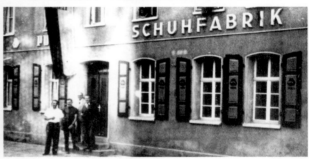

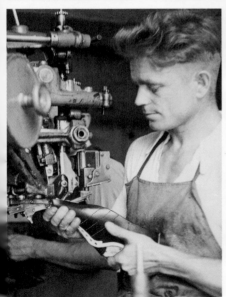

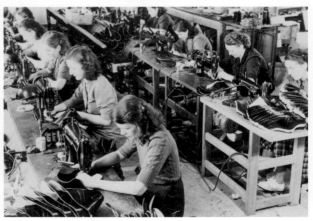

Puma's founder Rudolf Dassler with a young footballer, top left. The craft and innovation that the company brought to football-boot design and manufacture from the late 1940s soon gave it a reputation as a global leader in the field.

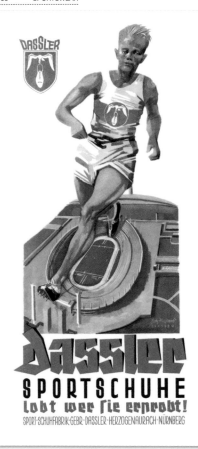

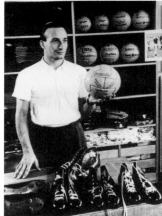

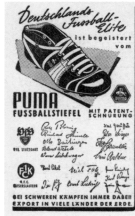

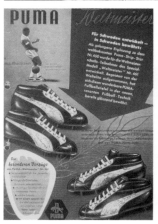

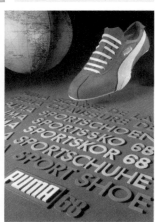

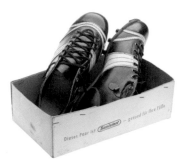

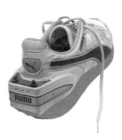

Puma's heritage as a sports brand lies with football of the post-war period, but by the 1960s the brand had extended to compete with Adidas (launched by the brother of Puma's founder) in the fields of athletics and tennis, with young champion Boris Becker lending his name to one of Puma's more covetable styles. Puma's sponsorship power became such that track star Linford Christie took the brand more literally to heart.

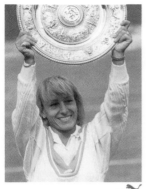

MARTINA NAVRATILOVA

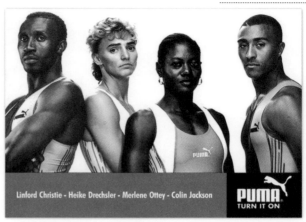

Linford Christie · Heike Drechsler · Merlene Ottey · Colin Jackson **PUMA** TURN IT ON

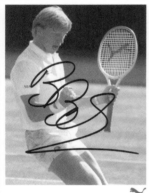

BORIS BECKER

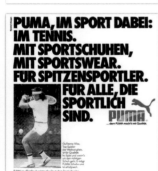

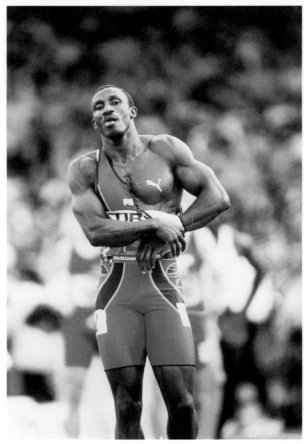

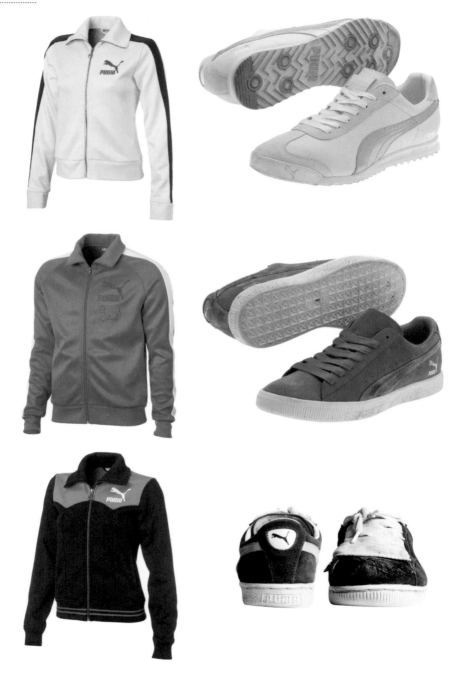

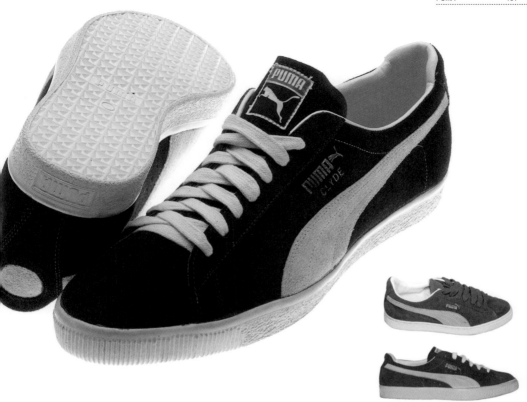

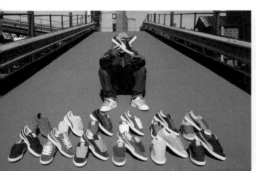

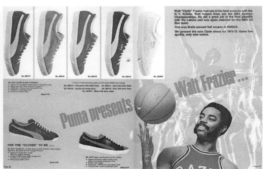

Puma's leaping big cat logo has found its way onto all kinds of sports kit, but its streetwear strength, in common with most sports brands, lies in its sneakers. Oddities have included styles with built-in training computers (see page 158, bottom right). Hits include Puma Roma, launched in 1968 but popular among British Casuals of the 1980s, and – perhaps king of Puma's sneakers – the Suede (1968) (opposite centre). The Suede was embraced by B-boys and updated as the Clyde, after the nickname given to dandy and basketball star Walt Frazier.

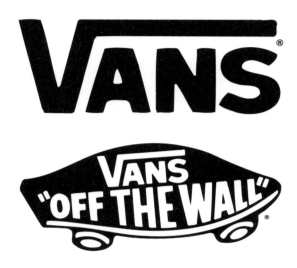

Vans' success, in part at least, was down to a lucky break. At the turn of the 1980s, a bored high-school kid apparently ripped the rubber off the side of his canvas shoes and started colouring in a checkerboard design. One of Vans' employees saw the design and suggested that the company run up some similar fabric. Then came a stroke of luck: a production company was looking for shoes for the cast of *Fast Times at Ridgemont High*, a teen movie starring an up-and-coming young actor called Sean Penn. Vans suddenly had a phenomenon on its hands and was having to make the style in every colour and combination it could think of.

The shoe style became known as the Checkerboard – a simple, slip-on sneaker, born out of California skate culture and adopted by edgier rock stars, art-student alternatives and middle-youth creatives, based on a model designed in 1966, just seven years after the first commercial skateboard, the Roller Derby Skateboard, hit the market. The southern California company behind the style, one of a handful of classics it has created, is the world's biggest skate shoe brand. But the company has humble roots in the mom-and-pop store attitude that saw founder Paul Van Doren work 20 years for Randy's, a Boston shoe company making canvas shoes for Boston Celtics players, before deciding to go it alone. His incentive? Randy's had sent him to California to whip its failing factory into shape – and in eight months it was doing better than the one back in Boston.

Success did not come overnight to the Van Doren Rubber Company, one of only four companies ever to make vulcanized rubber footwear in the US, alongside Randy's, Keds and Converse. Van Doren was so set on opening his own retail operation that for the first 10 years the company sold its minimalistic, old-fashioned back-to-basics sneakers to just 50 local stores. Indeed, it was because skateboard pioneers chose Vans, rather than Vans chasing them, that the company would become a streetwear icon and a company valued in hundreds of millions of dollars.

Here was not just a local company or one with growing ties to the then fledgling world of action sports, but one with (akin to the more East Coast brand Converse) an affordable, washable product that seemed designed for staying upright while performing an ollie or any other tricky skateboarding move. Even if it wasn't. The shoes were just tough: double thick rubber soles, heavyweight duck canvas, nylon, not cotton thread – "built like Sherman tanks" as Van Doren put it. This was a product with a DIY punk-rock aesthetic too and, inevitably, riders customized them.

Here was also a company that was even prepared to custom-make shoes – take in a piece of fabric, as riders from Manhattan Beach and Santa Monica would do, and Vans would do its best to colour-match it. It would even sell single shoes to allow for the fact that skateboarders would wear one shoe out faster than the other – in so doing, it began a trend for skaters to wear mismatched shoes deliberately. Vans also introduced a shoe with leather in the toe and heel, because that is where skaters wore them out fastest. Later came shoes with protective padded heels and ankles – notably the Skate Hi.

Skateboarding has made accessible for mainstream fashion the combat trouser, hoodie and wallet chain, the beanie hat and trucker cap, the outsize t-shirt and super-baggy jeans, each a street trend in its own right, each finding its origin in a skate park

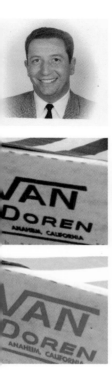

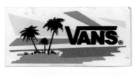

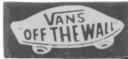

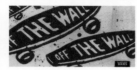

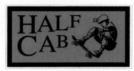

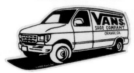

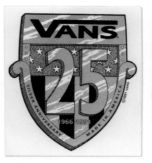

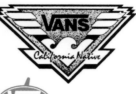

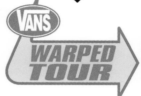

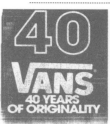

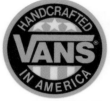

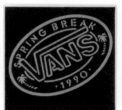

mewhere – and each invariably accompanied by a pair of Vans.
d it was to the first pro skaters that Vans first reached out: the
es of Tony Alva and Stacy Peralta – legendary, groundbreaking
ateboarders who adopted Vans' Era (skateboarding's first
ecially designed shoe back in 1976, incorporating the now
ndard necessities of grip, cushioning, good looks and,
reasingly, provenance) – as well as Steve Caballero, for whom
e company designed the first signature skate shoe. By 1977,
ns had its own skateboarding team, run by a man with a van
d a Plexiglass ramp. He would tour the skate spaces and make
re the best skaters got what he thought were the best shoes:
air of Vans.

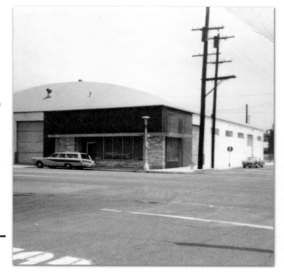

l Van Doren, Vans' founder, amid the many typographical treatments that the
tewear brand has undergone over the last few decades. Here, too, is the
nymous California factory from which a global brand was launched.

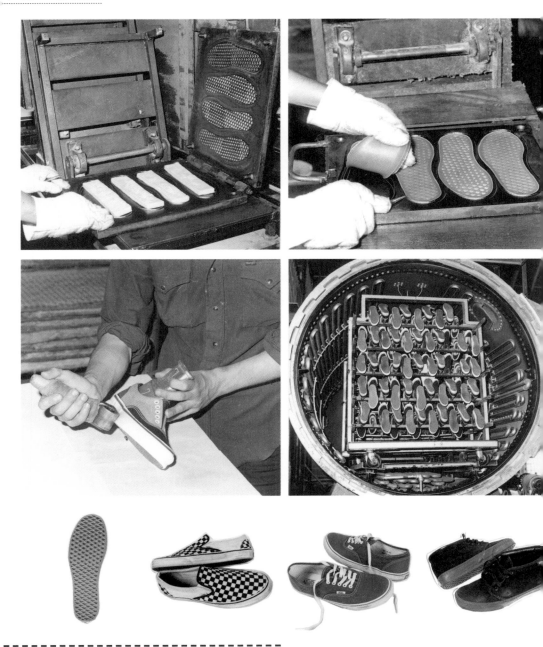

Laying, baking, gluing and trimming: the making of the super-tough but inexpensive vulcanized rubber sole that characterizes a Vans shoe, and which has made them so popular with skateboarders.

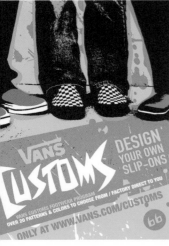

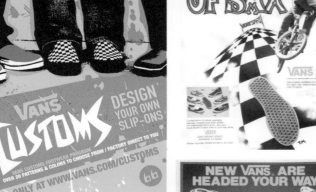

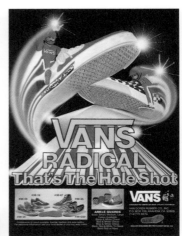

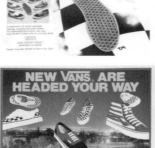

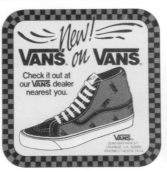

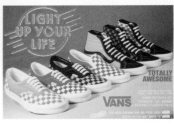

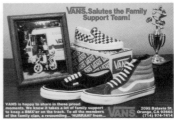

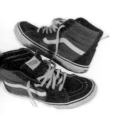

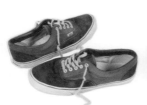

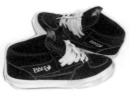

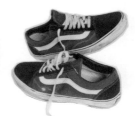

Skateboarding may have been the lynchpin of Vans' customer base, but Vans also won popularity during the breakdancing scene of the late 1970s and early 1980s and, more recently, with BMXers. Few of Vans' fashion designs have matched its most basic styles, notably the Checkerboard slip-on (bottom row second from left), Authentic (third from left), Half Cab (fourth) and Old Skool (far right).

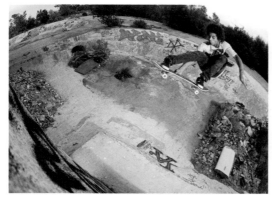
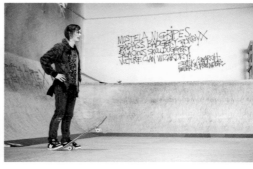
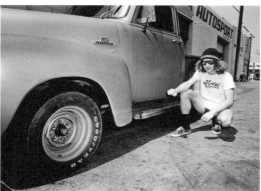
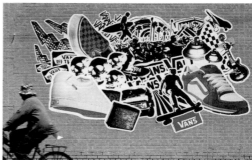
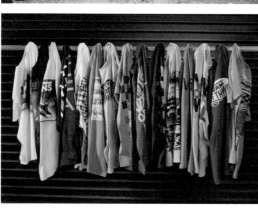
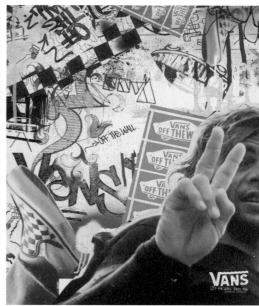

Vans has long established close ties with street cultures, whether skateboarding or graffiti writing – being a major sponsor of the former, and often co-opting the latter for advertising purposes. Above centre is skateboarding legend Tony Alva.

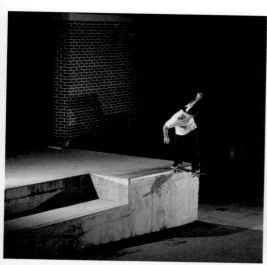
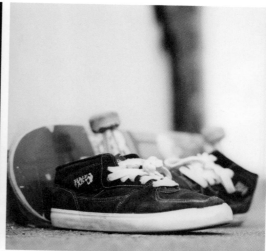
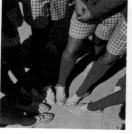
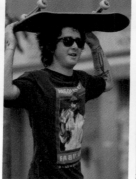
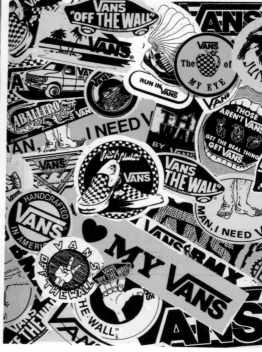
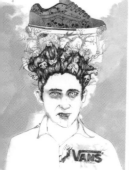
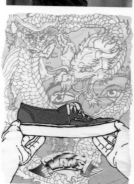

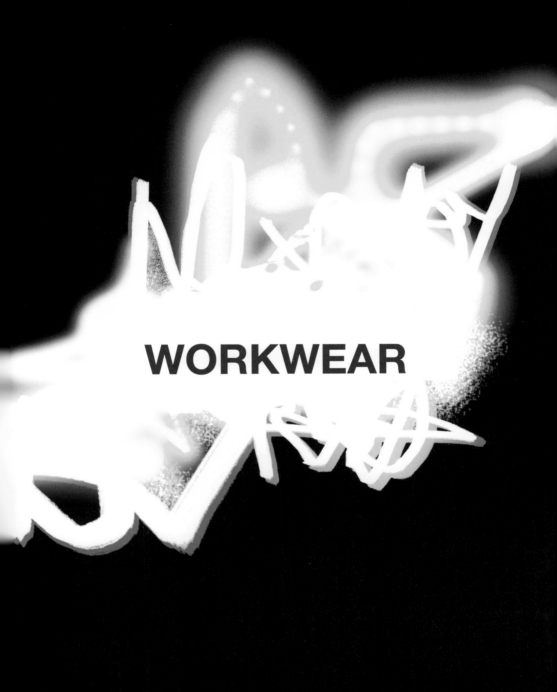

WORKWEAR

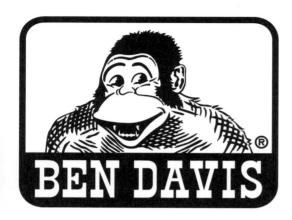

'Union Made. Plenty Tough.' Few tag-lines capture the spirit of workwear, if not streetwear, quite so eloquently – clothing made in the US and ready to take hard knocks. This was the simple aspiration of Benjamin Franklin Davis, a survivor of the era's economic meltdown who, in 1935, aged just 21, set up a business to supply the man anxious that his clothing goes the distance. The move was born of sheer necessity. "In those days we were in severe depression and you had to work to make a living," Ben Davis explained. "If you didn't make a living you starved to death. I was playing professional saxophone at the time. We had a three-piece combo. In those days almost everyone danced and the radio was not good and records were no good either, so we got jobs almost every Saturday night. We played all over but you still couldn't make a living. My father knew some people who had some money in a roughly similar garment business, and he persuaded them to set up this business and I ran it. I eventually bought out those people and that was the end of it."

Not quite. The company is still family-owned, and run by Ben's son, Frank Davis – "I guess you could say clothes manufacturing is in the blood," he noted. But it has latterly found a demand supplying the man whose work is less arduous and who just wants to look good. In part this is down to the company's recognition of streetwear as a market, launching a specialist line, along with a skateboard tour. But it is also because streetwear, especially on the West Coast of the US, has embraced the loose comfort and sturdy fabrics of the original clothing, still cut using patterns first drawn up in the 1930s.

Key to the operation have been the Original trouser, a wide-legged pair of trousers with popper-button slit pockets to the rear and frog-mouth pockets to the front (with the supersized 'gorilla cut' pants a perfect fit for baggy street style); and the short-sleeved, zip-up pull-over shirt – a modified version of a pattern bought by Ben Davis from Neustadter Bros., a now defunct company that made what it called the 'Boss of the Road' shirt. Fans have included the Beastie Boys, Ice Cube and, perhaps above all, rapper Dr. Dre, all of whom have rapped about the brand. In one video Dr. Dre is seen deciding what shirt to wear – in front of a closet full only of black Ben Davis shirts.

"Working clothes are generally not a high style item – it's more of a basic thing," Frank Davis said. "One group called us asking us to make them some XXXXX large shirts. Some of these guys like to wear this big, big, big, way oversized stuff."

The brand's high visibility has also been enhanced by its cheeky simian logo – fortunately, a perfect graphic device for t-shirts and one that has been widely imitated by other streetwear brands. X-Large, SSUR and A Bathing Ape are among those who have, perhaps in homage, perhaps out of an enduring fascination with films such as *Planet of the Apes*, *2001: A Space Odyssey* and other examples of 1970s pop culture, also adopted ape logos. Ben Davis's explanation for its use is far more prosaic: "In those days [the 1930s onwards] there were a number of firms making similar merchandise. There was one that had a rooster for a logo, one that had a bulldog [the aforementioned Neustadter Bros.], one with the headlamp of a locomotive and so forth. I conceived the idea of putting in the ape or gorilla. I had a professional artist draw three of them and I picked the best of the three. Other apes have been biting my banana for years."

The history behind Ben Davis, however, is far longer and lies truly at the heart of the workwear that underpins so much streetwear. It was the 1870s and a woman was visiting a tailor in Reno, Nevada, established by one Jacob Davis, a Latvian – and Ben Davis's grandfather – who had emigrated to San Francisco in the 1860s and had since made a living making not just work clothes to outfit those mining in the great gold rush, but also tents and horse blankets, made from duck, a thick cotton fabric, and reinforced with copper rivets. The female customer was trying to find some cheap trousers for her large husband, who wore through them at an unreasonable rate.

Having noticed that thread alone often did not prevent pockets coming off his garments – given the unforgiving use to which they were put, carrying heavy tools – Davis decided this was the opportunity to experiment. He applied rivets to all the stress points on the trousers and, never hearing from the woman again, could well assume that they stood up to her husband's endurance test. By the following year Davis was riveting all of the trousers he made and had even applied for a patent, which was approved in 1873 and which he held until it expired in 1908.

The man who helped Davis apply for the patent? His fabric supplier, one Levi Strauss, the pioneer of denim jeans. Indeed, Davis spent the rest of that century and up to 1908 living in San Francisco and overseeing production of riveted trousers at the Valencia Street factory of Levi Strauss and Company. "The secratt of them Pants is the Rivits that I put in those Pockots and I found the demand so large that I cannot make them fast enough," Davis

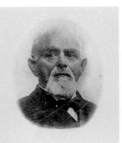
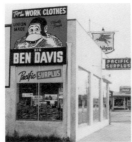
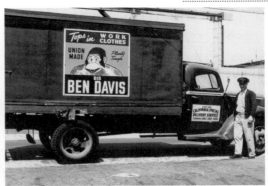
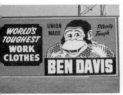
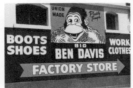
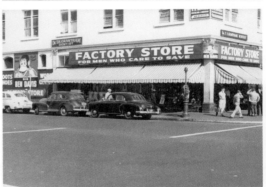

rote, in semi-literate English, to Strauss. "My nabors are getting
ealouse of these success and unless I secure it by Patent Papers
will soon become to be a general thing everybody will make
em up and thare will be no money in it."

  With Davis offering Strauss "half the right to sell all such
lothing Revited" in certain US territories in return for covering
alf the cost of filing the patent, it was Strauss who would go
n to make the fortune, with the rivet an integral part of his now
onic five-pocket western jeans. "He [Jacob Davis] had a number
f children. He wanted to patent the idea of the pocket rivet. His
ife, my grandmother, protested because it would have cost $75
o make the patent, money that they did not have – they needed
t for food for the children," Ben Davis explained. Nowadays,
onically perhaps, Ben Davis clothes do not come riveted. But
ey are still plenty tough.

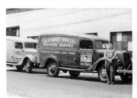
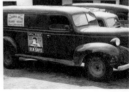
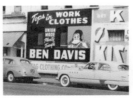
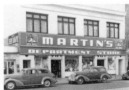
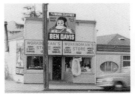
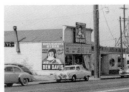

acob Davis (top left), grandfather of the brand and creator of the rivet that helped
ake the name of one Levi Strauss & Co. Ben Davis himself may not have become
 big name, but in the years before the Second World War Ben Davis branded pants
nd shirts could be found in almost every town across the US.

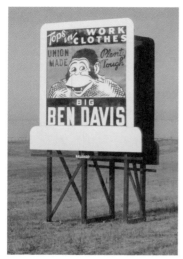

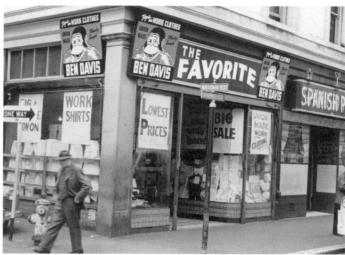

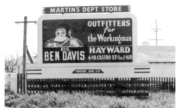

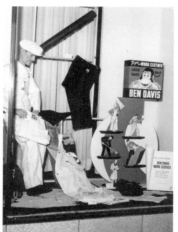

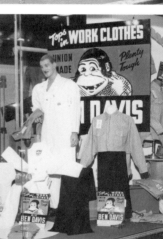

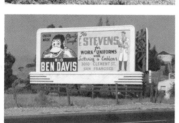

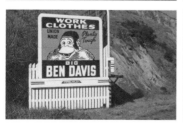

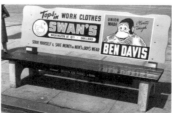

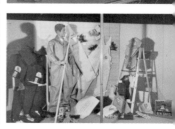

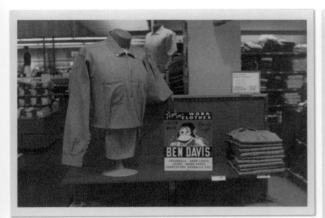

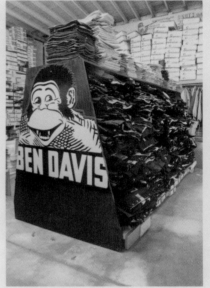

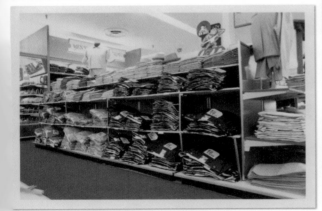

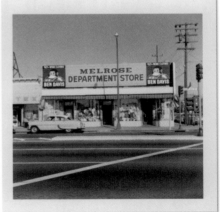

Ben Davis was once a definitive and certainly ubiquitous workwear brand – 'outfitters for the Workingman', as one hoarding has it – and advertised extensively, on railway platforms, alongside freeways, in shop windows and across park benches. The brand has never promoted itself as fashionable, as the pile-it-high approach of its in-store displays suggests.

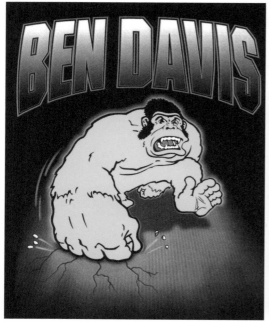

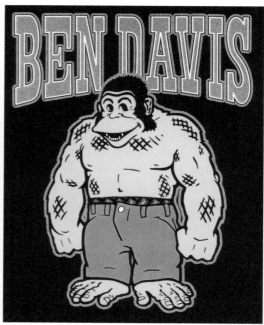

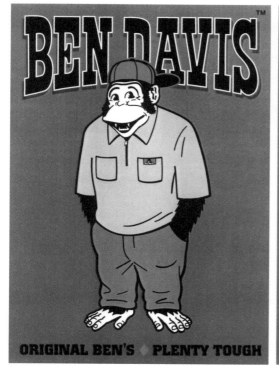

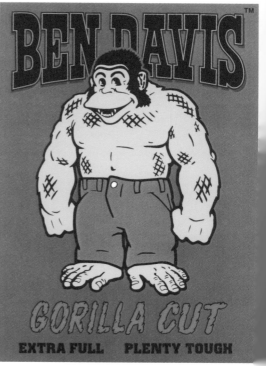

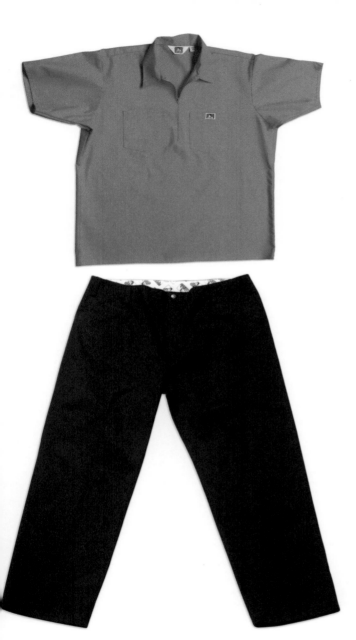

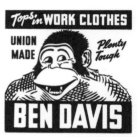

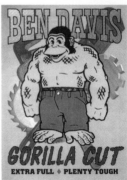

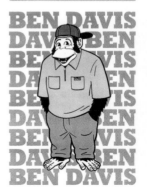

...e ape – Ben Davis's chosen symbol of strength and endurance – was not only widely imitated in the decades ...mediately after the brand's launch, by boot company Gorilla Shoe among others, but has been imitated more ...ensively since the 1990s, with A Bathing Ape the most obvious example. The influence of the Ben Davis logo ...s been extensive in relation to that of its products. While Ben Davis also makes overalls, it has achieved cult ...tus with just two now classic garments: its Original pants and the half-zipper front short-sleeved shirt.

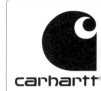

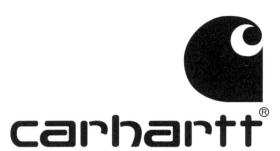

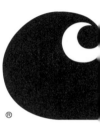

Carhartt is a severe case of schizophrenia for the fashion world. On the one hand, the business's European operation is run (alongside 'industrialwear' and 'workwear' divisions) as a leading streetwear brand, with Carhartt recognized as a source of tough, well-built basics (supplemented by clever graphics and occasional bold colour) by skaters, BMXers and those who like the look. On the other hand, this version of Carhartt would leave an American customer nonplussed: in its home market, it remains one of the original workwear companies. Worn by men on construction sites, it is a brand that has stayed close to its roots – strictly hardware rather than streetwear.

This, of course, lends the brand a certain, esteemed authenticity. Carhartt's first product was a pioneering overall garment designed specifically for railroad workers, based on discussions with railway engineers. This was more than an attempt to buck competition by making products that were different – although that possibility certainly occurred to the brand's entrepreneurial founder, Hamilton Carhart, who was born in Macedon Lock, New York, in 1855 and grew up in southern Michigan. It was he, after all, who decided that adding an extra 't' to his surname would make it more memorable. His first line of work was in a furnishing business, but that chance conversation with the railroad employee sparked the realization that the new breed of industrial worker behind the country's transport and building boom needed clothes fit for purpose. Until this point, the clothing of blue-collar workers was worn as much for leisure as for hard graft. "I believe that when a man wears an article that I manufacture, his self-respect is increased because he knows that it is made by an honest manufacturer, who is honest with his employees," Carhartt once stated.

The story of the eponymous company Hamilton Carhartt, established in 1889, is, however, one of small beginnings: overalls made from duck and denim fabrics by five employees sharing four sewing machines, with Carhartt pressing the flesh at railroads across the US to build a workable customer base. But, finding a niche, the company grew as rapidly as the great US cities themselves – and was just as badly hit by the Great Depression,

which left only three of 17 factories and three mills in operation in the country after 1930. But Carhartt, as might be expected, bounced back, consolidating his business with the opening of new headquarters in Irvine, Kentucky – where they remain today, still a family-owned business – and, with his 'Back to the Land' campaign, building a new market with agricultural workers. By the time Carhartt died in 1937, aged 82, his brand was established as the market leader in the new category of workwear and the company motto, 'from the mill to millions', was being fulfilled. The company operated its own cotton production, denim mills and manufacturing plants, with fabrics such as its 'master cloth', setting an industry benchmark; its designs, including its mountain coat, double-knee pants and carpenter pants – with their distinctive side-seam tool pocket and belt loops – were copied widely. Products for the oil and gas industries and fire services followed. Need a character to look especially rugged? Carhartt has featured in movies as diverse, and as macho, as *Training Day*, *Armageddon*, *Jurassic Park* and *War of the Worlds*.

Need it to work for the streetwear market, however? In 1994 the German company Work in Progress, Carhartt's European distributor, adapted the brand with a collection better suited both to more youth-oriented and European customers, quickly establishing Carhartt as a streetwear staple – not only for the functionality of its clothing, but through association with the wider scene. Carhartt has, for example, been a regular sponsor of the European Skateboard Championships, run its own pro skateboard and BMX teams (and sold its own BMX cruiser), co-designed special items with the likes of Burton Snowboards, Vans and Honda, and collaborated for its advertising campaigns with recognized street artists such as Won ABC, Mode 2 and Belgian illustrator Dave Decat.

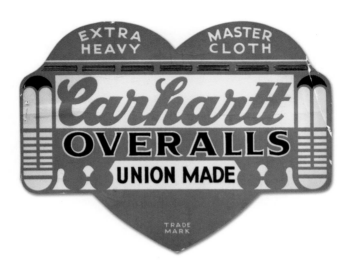

Although co-opted as a streetwear brand in the European market, Carhartt's labelling has always stressed its durability and functionality: 'extra heavy', 'built right', 'as rugged as the men who wear them'. These are clothes as tools, but they also show the graphic potential that is the lynchpin of streetwear design.

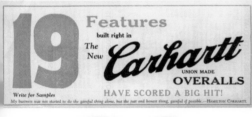

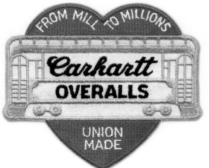

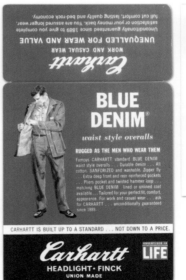

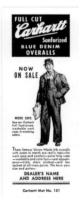

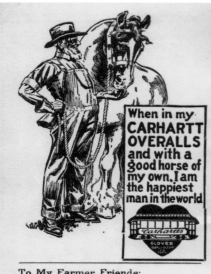

When in my
**CARHARTT
OVERALLS**
and with a
good horse of
my own, I am
the happiest
man in the world

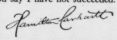

To My Farmer Friends:
  I have made it a part of my life to think always of the best, work for the best and expect the best; so when I began to manufacture overalls I was out to make garments of character that would bind customers to me with hooks of steel. Can you say I have not succeeded.

Hamilton Carhartt

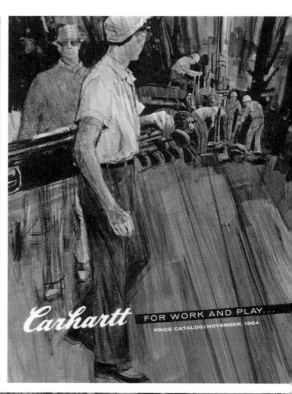

Carhartt FOR WORK AND PLAY...
PRICE CATALOG/NOVEMBER, 1964

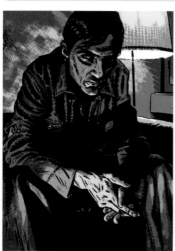

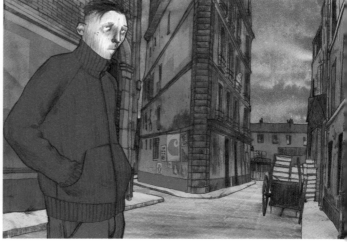

Carhartt has maintained the ethos of its original advertising – often simple and illustrative – in more recent campaigns, working with distinctive and collectible illustrators, among them Benjamin Gudel (above left and opposite top row), Mode2 (opposite bottom row) and Dave Decat (above right and opposite middle row).

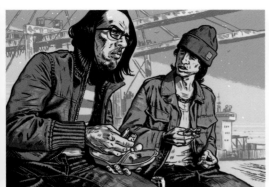
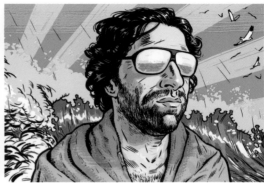
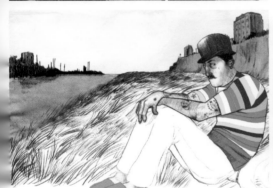
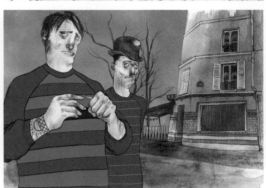
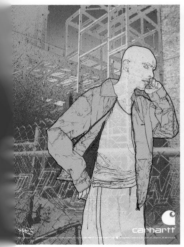
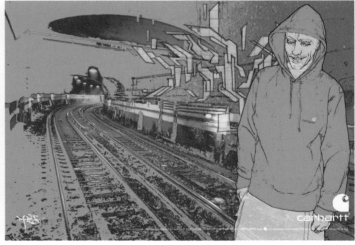

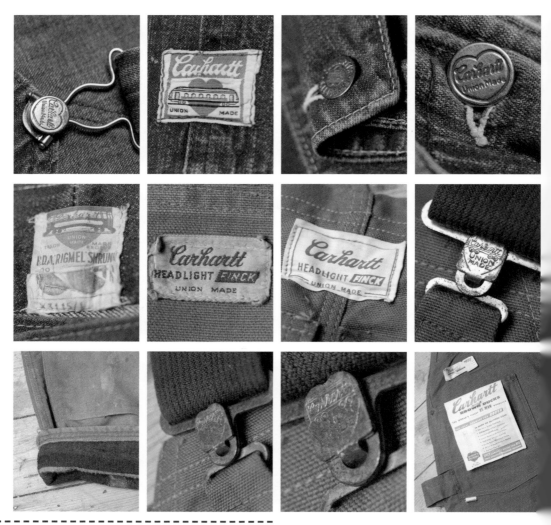

The other side of Carhartt. While the brand has an established following as a streetwear label, its origins are in functional workwear, from chore and hunting jackets to overalls and dungarees, many made from the tough tan-coloured canvas fabric, a precursor to denim, known as duck.

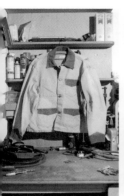
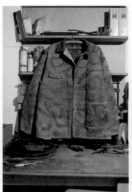
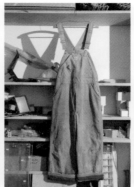
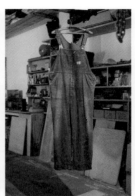

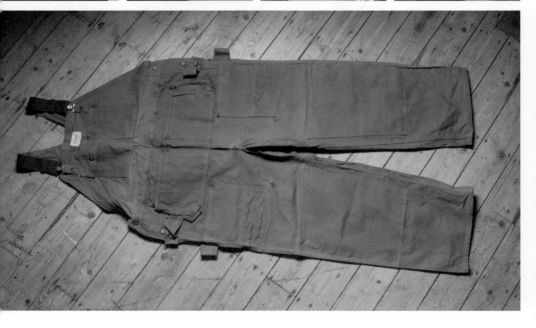

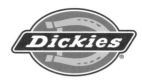

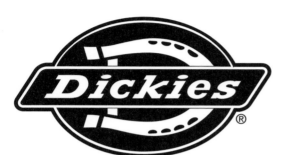

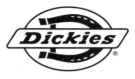

When skaters want to dress up, they put on a pair of Dickies 874s. Of course, the dressing up is relative – but as an alternative to jeans, these flat-fronted poly-cotton trousers, with a permanent crease, were designed to make American working men presentable when dealing with the public. It was a uniform that was hard-wearing, quick-drying and always crisp. A blend of functionality and style made the 874 a classic, although skaters often prefer Dickies' baggier Double-Knee Work Pants, for obvious reasons. The brand's appeal to the streetwear market has also been considerably enhanced by its logo, whose 1950s type and side-on horseshoe (a nod to the company's origins as harness-makers) are fashionable in their own right.

Skaters may not have been the intended market for a company that went on to produce coveralls, high-visibility garments, flame-retardant jackets, lab coats and foul-weather outerwear, not to mention workwear for the likes of Shell, Volkswagen, JCB and John Deere. But Dickies conceded its fashion appeal in the early 2000s with the launch of a series of street-art sponsorship programmes and its own streetwear line, albeit one that, unusually, meets international safety standards. Yet, as the company's publicity material expresses it, "Where does stylish workwear end and practical streetwear begin in today's world of harmonized boundaries?"

Dickies' youth appeal (not to mention its adoption during the 1990s by neo-punkish 'skater bands' such as Limp Bizkit, Blink 182, Green Day, No Doubt and Avril Lavigne) would undoubtedly have perplexed C. N. Williamson and E. E. 'Colonel' Dickie of Bryan, Texas, who in 1918 decided to downscale their 'vehicle and harness' business and launch the U.S. Overall Company, ready to feed America's post-war industrial boom. Four years later, C. Don Williamson joined with his father and cousin to buy the company, renaming it the Williamson-Dickie Manufacturing Company, from

which came the Dickies brand and a reputation for making hard-wearing kit. Given that 'Colonel' Dickie was bought out of the company, why the Dickies rather than a Williamson brand name was subsequently born remains a mystery.

With the exception of the years preceding the Great Depression that began in the late 1920s, Dickies saw continued growth. Indeed, it was really the Second World War that made the company – it was sequestered by the US Government to make uniforms for the armed services. This also launched them into classic films – Frank Sinatra, in uniform, wears Dickies in *From Here to Eternity* (1953). With profits from the war it was possible to increase manufacturing capacity and supply decent, dependable clothing to millions of men. This reaffirmed the company's credibility, as well as built it a reputation, and was a key step toward making Dickies the world's largest manufacturer of workwear, now based out of Fort Worth, Texas. A second piece of good fortune also assisted the company in its growth – during their travels to strike deals overseas, Texan oilmen introduced Dickies to oilfield workers in the Middle East.

Dickies has certainly not ditched its workwear heritage in order to chase the fashion buck – fashion has come to it. The company became the key sponsor of the little-known Worker of the Year contest, in which the winner gets a weekend in Nashville and takes home … what else but a new Dodge Ram pick-up truck?

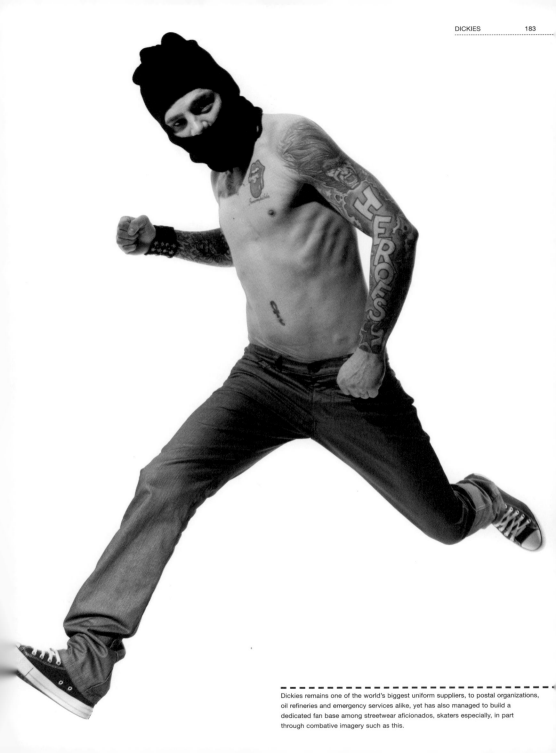

Dickies remains one of the world's biggest uniform suppliers, to postal organizations, oil refineries and emergency services alike, yet has also managed to build a dedicated fan base among streetwear aficionados, skaters especially, in part through combative imagery such as this.

For the street and of the street – Dickies' advertising has long captured its products in situ, worn by mechanics, cycle couriers, tattooists: ordinary people needing extraordinarily tough clothing.

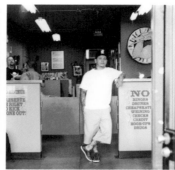
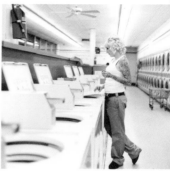

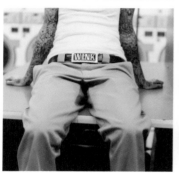
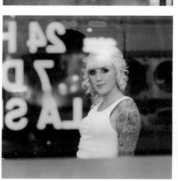
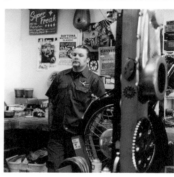

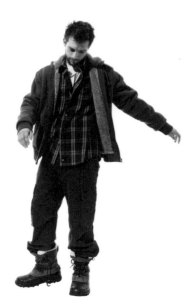
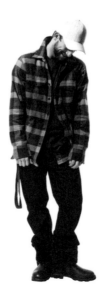
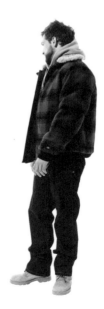

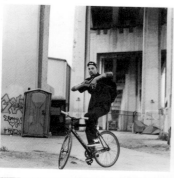
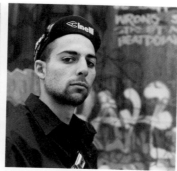
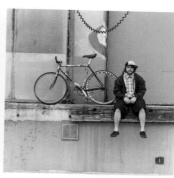
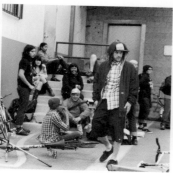
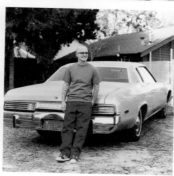
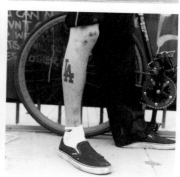

Streetwear from the likes of Dickies has always kept its blue-collar roots and regard for the functional clothing required by outdoorsmen, hunters and loggers, even if the appreciation is more stylistic than practical.

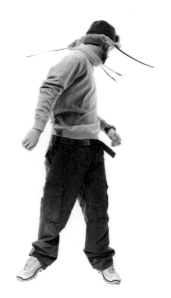
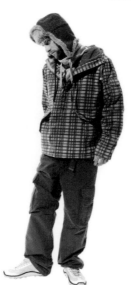
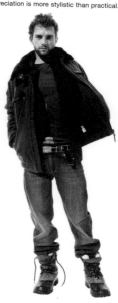

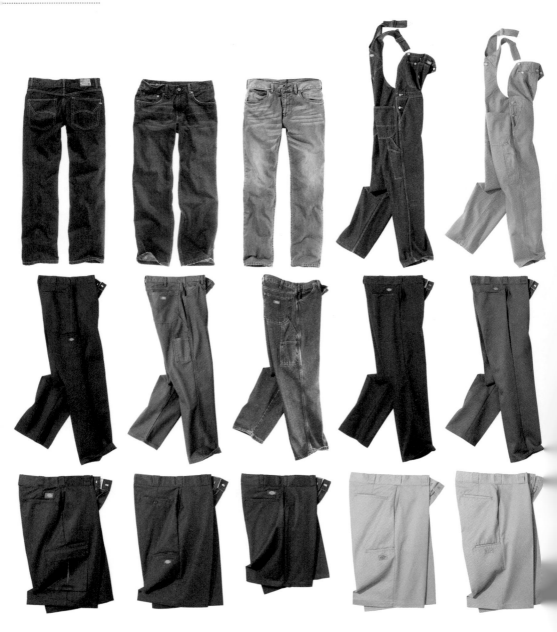

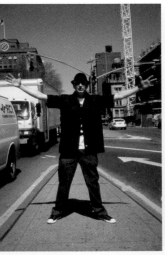 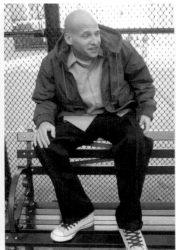 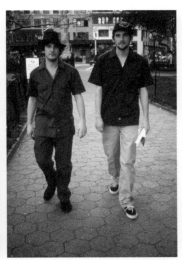

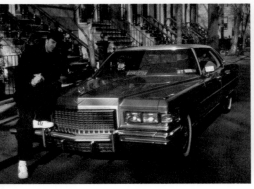 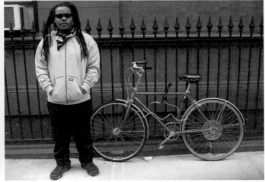

ckies may make traditional five-pocket western jeans, but its reputation stands on
e crisp, poly-cotton 874 styles, opposite centre row right, which lend even skaters
smarter look. The shirt, top left, is typically worn outsized and short-sleeved,
metimes over a long-sleeved undershirt.

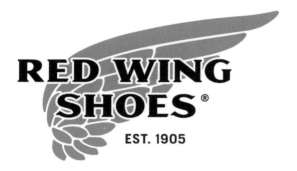

That a shaggy, country breed of dog should give the name to an iconic piece of workwear adopted by the urban streetwear market may provide a touch of irony. But the Irish Setter work boot, with its white sole and its reddish leather mimicking the distinctive coat of the upland bird dog (pointer or setter), was always more than just a boot: it has been consistently representative of the classic Americana that, along with dark, baggy denims, wallet chains and tough outerwear, has maintained a lasting, albeit niche, subsection of the streetwear scene. The boot – as with workwear in general – was a counter to the dressier, preppy style provided by the likes of Ralph Lauren: this was genuine blue-collar territory, a statement of being separate from, rather than seeking in any way to emulate, white-collar chic, even among those who had never been down a mine or worked in a railway yard. As such, the authenticity of the product was essential – and Red Wing had it.

The company was started in 1905, by a German immigrant, Charles Beckman, much like the legendary workwear pioneer Levi Strauss. Beckman named the company after the local town of just 16,000 people, set in the bluffs of the Mississippi River. The town was named after the Dakota Tribe's Chief Red Wing, a title handed down through the generations; the son of the very first Chief Red Wing was called Tatankamani, a Dakota word meaning, appropriately for a boot company, 'Walking Buffalo'. The Minnesota territory made a welcome market for hard-wearing boots: the region comprised huge forests, farmlands and iron mines, all subject to extremes of weather, searing heat in the summer but bitter, sub-zero temperatures in the winter. With heavy industry also in expansion, Red Wing boots found a ready market, most notably for its Brown Chief farmer's model of 1919, the predecessor of the Irish Setter. With war, it found an even more buoyant market: during the First World War, Red Wing supplied the US Army with its 'No. 16' boots; they were also issued during the Second World War, when they were available in 239 different sizes and widths to ensure comfort on long marches.

But it wasn't until the 1950s and early 1960s – the classic era of Americana to which 'retro' trends most frequently return – that the Red Wing became a popular leisure boot across the US, seemingly designed to look just so with jeans. Perhaps nothing could drive this point home more forcefully today than the fact that the advertising images of the time were drawn by Norman Rockwell, whose hard-working, hard-playing, red-cheeked characters, straight from Main Street, have helped define the era in the popular imagination.

The Red Wing boot might have an even firmer place in street culture's history if it wasn't for a costume designer giving way to an actor. Harrison Ford was slated to wear a pair of Red Wings in his role as Indiana Jones in Steven Spielberg's *Raiders* film franchise. But Ford suggested an alternative: the boots (made by another US bootmaker, Alden) that he had worn when he was working as a carpenter. That boot may now be known as the 'Indy', but still can't claim the more rugged street style appreciated in the Red Wing.

Charles Beckman, the German immigrant who founded Red Wing (opposite top left) and his factory. The company is named, like the town in which it was established, after the historic Native American chief of the area.

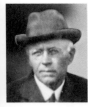

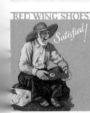

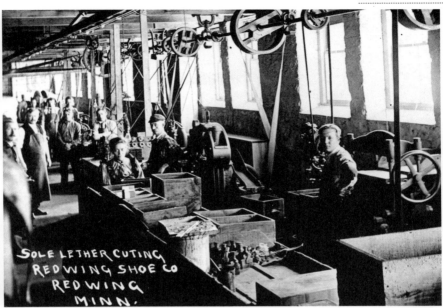

SOLE LETHER CUTING
REDWING SHOE CO
REDWING
MINN.

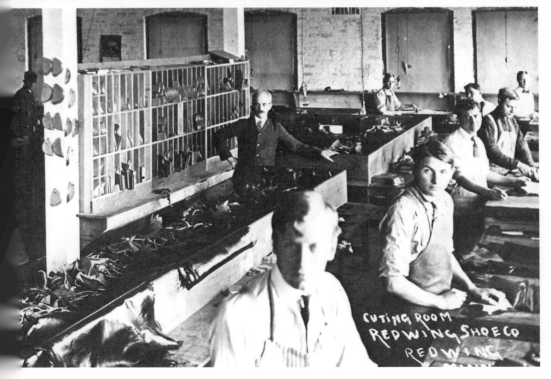

CUTING ROOM
REDWING SHOE CO
REDWING

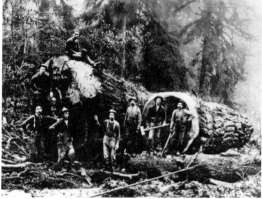
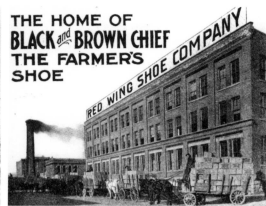

THE HOME OF
BLACK and BROWN CHIEF
THE FARMER'S
SHOE

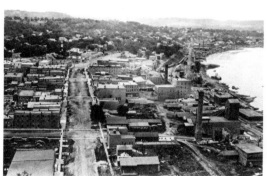
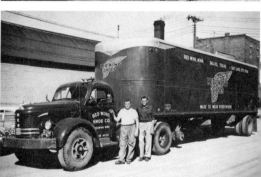

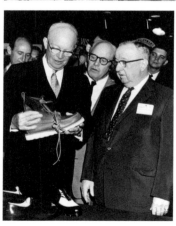
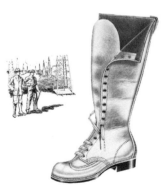
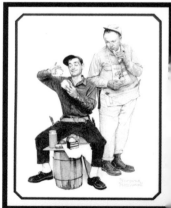

Loggers at work in Red Wings (top left), and below them the town of Red Wing. Red
Wings became so much an established part of American culture that they drew the
attention of President Eisenhower and (bottom row right), the illustrations of Norman
Rockwell, which defined the image of the American blue-collar working man during
the 1940s and 1950s.

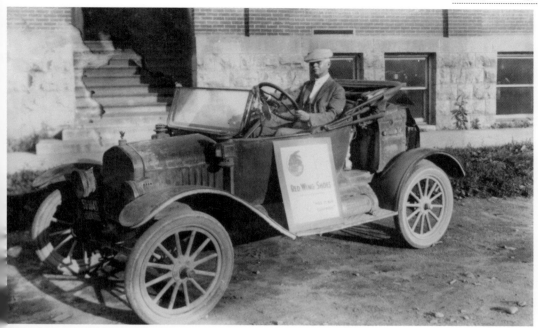

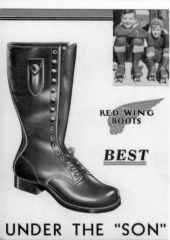

RED WING BOOTS

BEST

UNDER THE "SON"

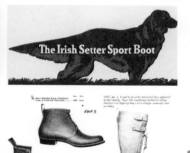

The Irish Setter Sport Boot

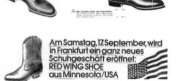

Am Samstag, 17. September, wird in Frankfurt ein ganz neues Schuhgeschäft eröffnet: RED WING SHOE aus Minnesota/USA

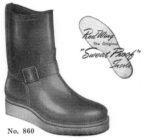

Red Wing The Original "Sweat-Proof" Insole

No. 860

- ● UPPERS   9-inch Setter Red Oro Russet, Wellington type boot, leather lined vamp
- ● INSOLE   "SWEAT-PROOF" leather, will not crack
- ● SOLE   Cushion Crepe, light and long wearing, nail-less construction, all around sewed welt
- ● HEEL   Cushion Crepe wedge, all around sewed heel seat
- ● COUNTER   Heavy leather

Width	6	½	7	½	8	½	9	½	10	½	11	½	12	½	13
C		x	x	x	x	x	x	x	x	x	x	x	x		x
E	x	x	x	x	x	x	x	x	x		x	x	x	x	x

Salesmen travelled coast to coast from the 1910s promoting Red Wings as the definitive working footwear to farmers, ranch-hands and the new heavy industries. Advanced production techniques saw Red Wing become a major local employer.

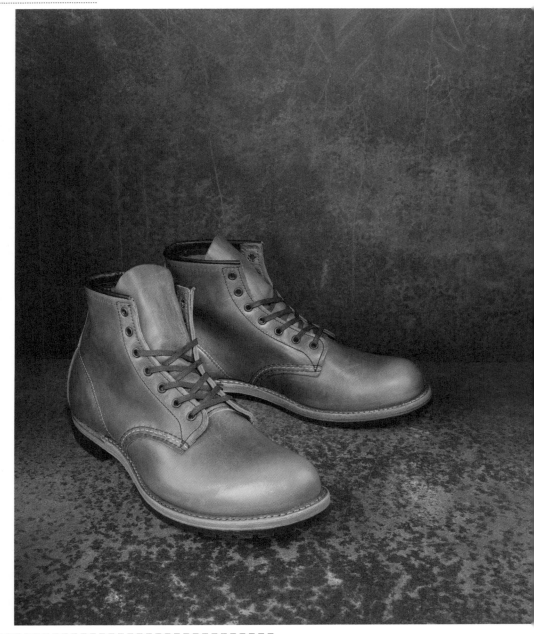

Many of Red Wing's sales have been those of contemporary styles – hiker and
sneaker hybrids, for example. But the company also recognizes the appeal of its
Depression-era styles. One reissue is this, its Gentleman Traveller, originally designed
for door-to-door salesmen walking long distances but needing to look smart.

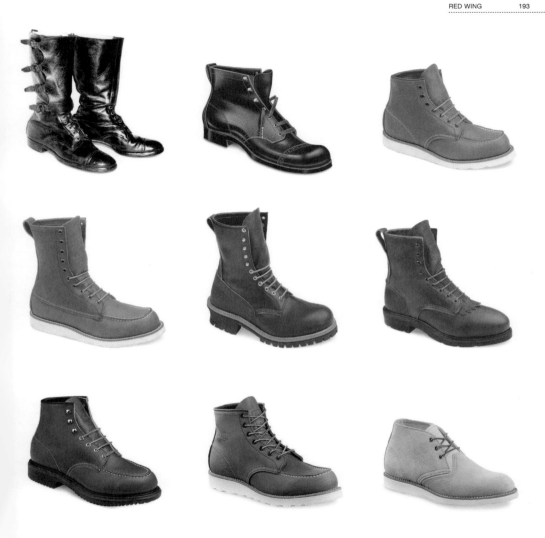

Red Wing's boots, old and new, show the evolution of a basic style with upper and sole designed with a specific wearer in mind, among them biker, logger, oilman. Among classic styles, uppers have barely changed for a century, with most technical advances seen in the soles, from leather towards oil- and chemical-resistant synthetic composites, most notably the distinctive white sole of the Irish Setter style (bottom row centre).

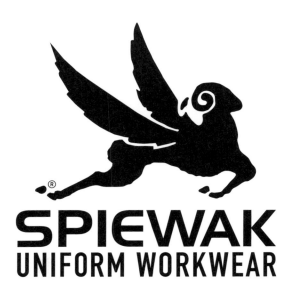

The streetwear market was not one that Spiewak had intended entering. Workwear, yes; specialist outerwear items for the military too; even, inexplicably given that it had no heritage in the market, deciding in 1979 that it would spend the next decade making cowboy clothes. But when in 1995 rap group Junior Mafia wore Spiewak EMS in a shoot for one of the first issues of the influential hip-hop magazine *The Source*, it found itself fuelling a new fashion interest in technical workwear, albeit one that Japanese youth had discovered when the company launched there in 1976.

Within two years of *The Source* giving Spiewak a new spin, its own brand was not only in the ascendant, but it was making authentic outerwear for many other urban brands – Stussy, Supreme, Phat Farm and the Wu-Tang Clan's own brand among them – and was being worn by rappers such as Biggie Smalls and Jay-Z. Business doubled in just a few years. A decade later it would be co-designing updated M-43 field jackets with the likes of Kidrobot.

But this was new ground for the brand. Like many US workwear companies, I. Spiewak and Sons began close to the turn of the 20th century, in 1904, with a singular product – in this case, sheepskin gilets (sleeveless jackets), which were big at the time. Isaac Spiewak, an immigrant from Poland, made his items in one room in Williamsburg, Brooklyn, New York, selling them himself at Red Hook Piers to dockers. His son Philip, who joined the company aged 15, brought in Fordist, streamlined, time-and-motion production methods – a pioneering move in clothing manufacture and one that helped the company weather the Depression of the late 1920s and beyond. All six of Isaac's sons were working for the company, or spin-offs of it, by the end of the 1930s (by the 1950s, Philip's three sons would also be working for Spiewak).

By then the company was well known for its Golden Fleece line of sheepskins, and its logo, a flying ram, had stuck. But, similar to Dickies, Red Wing and others, it benefited particularly from the boon to such businesses brought by two world wars and the consequent huge government contracts, most prominently, in Spiewak's case, to supply the US Navy during the Second World War with sheepskin flying suits, B-15 bomber jackets, Navy pea coats and N-1 deck jackets.

It was a boom time that continued because Spiewak launched itself as a brand with retail presence, and also because the fashion for utility or military-type garments (the bomber jacket especially) continued through the late 1940s and 1950s, prefiguring streetwear's interest in such items by some four decades. Demobbed soldiers, having grown used to their functionality during war service, found a role for them in civilian life. 'Wherever you go, whatever you do', as one Spiewak magazine advertisement put it at the time, stressing the brand's credentials as makers of highly functional clothing. This was the era in which Spiewak created a number of influential outerwear designs, among them the so-called Swiss Blouse and the Parbuster golf jacket.

Of course, Spiewak (as well as fellow military-inspired, American family-run companies, such as Schott) helped this along – creating the perfect market for all of its military surplus. But, atypically among workwear brands, Spiewak has maintained many of its wartime contracts, and still makes garments for military, police and specialist use, including Arctic expeditions, uniforms for the ground crews of American Airlines (a contract Spiewak has held since 1954) and kit for some 8,000 agencies worldwide.

Garments such as these may require a high degree of modern functionality, but the company, still in family hands, with Isaac's great-grandsons Michael and Roy Spiewak the latest generation

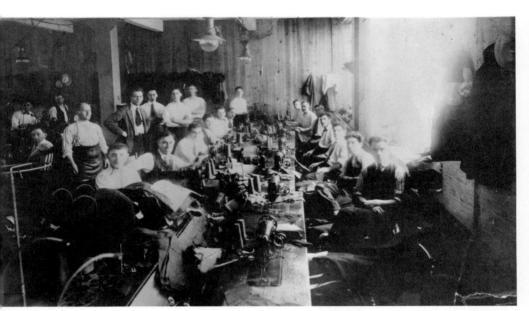

arge, makes full use of its extensive archive in developing
thing for both its Uniform Workwear and Street divisions. And it
s driven one or two of its own fads along the way: children of
1970s may recall the craze for the Snorkel parka, a Spiewak
del based on a traditional Inuit coat and originally designed for
US Air Force.

"Fashion came our way. We're trying to capitalize on that," as
chael Spiewak explained. "We used to say that if it's ugly and
worn outdoors, it's ours. Now we say if it's ugly and it's worn
doors, it's fashion, and it's still ours. But [unlike many fashion
npanies] we can be a successful brand without letting image
ertake the product. I look in the mirror every day and I know
nmy Hilfiger I'm not."

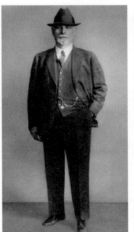

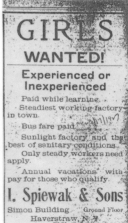

GIRLS
WANTED!
Experienced or
Inexperienced

Paid while learning.
Steadiest working factory
in town.

Bus fare paid.

Sunlight factory and the
best of sanitary conditions.

Only steady workers need
apply.

Annual vacations with
pay for those who qualify.

I. Spiewak & Sons
Simon Building   Ground Floor
Haverstraw, N. Y.

The Spiewak workshop was founded by Isaac Spiewak to make sheepskin coats,
much like those in the advertisement over the page. Spiewak's ad for help wanted
was more legitimate than it might seem at first glance.

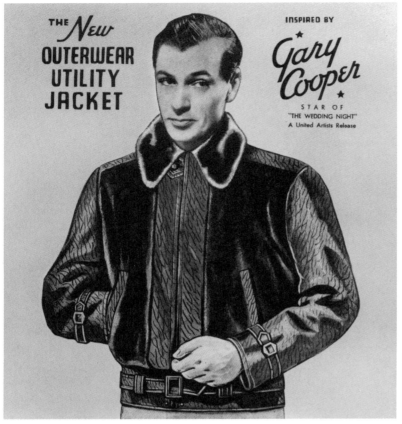

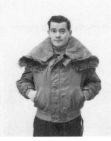

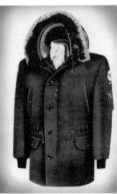

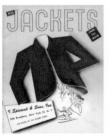

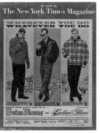

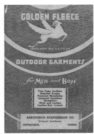

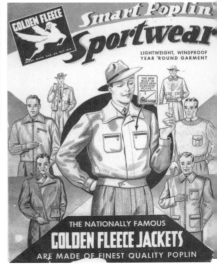

Advertisements from Spiewak's archives highlight the range of key styles it produced
– many from its top-of-the-range Golden Fleece line – which are still in production
today. Actor and style leader of his time Gary Cooper's endorsement would have
ensured considerable sales.

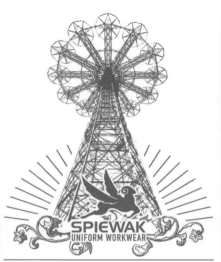

SPIEWAK
UNIFORM WORKWEAR

fred segal man   barneys co-op   american rag
www.spiewak.com

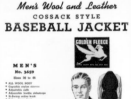
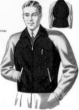
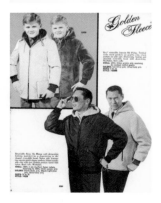
MENS SHEEPLINED COATS

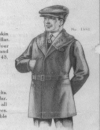

No. 1880 - 32-inch SHEEPLINED MOLESKIN COAT
(With 2 Pockets)
(See illustration on left)
Made of medium weight drab moleskin cloth; lined with selected sheepskin pelts. Sleeve lining made of warm, durable cloth. Has deep beaverized sheepskin collar. Fitted with woolen wristlets in sleeves. Has two slash pockets reinforced with leather. Closes with buttons and loops in double breasted style. Length 32 inches. Sizes 36 to 48.

No. 1883 - SHEEPLINED MOLESKIN COAT
(34 in., 2 Pockets and Belt)
Made of medium weight drab moleskin cloth; lined with heavy sheepskin pelts. Sleeve lining made of strong heavy cloth. Has wide collar of beaverized sheepskins. Warm woolen wristlets in sleeves. Has two slash pockets, reinforced with leather. Closes with buttons and loops in popular double breasted style. Has a broad belt all around with tongueless metal button. Length 34 inches. Sizes 36 to 48.

No. 1881 - 36-inch SHEEPLINED MOLESKIN COAT
(With 4 Pockets and Belt)
(See illustration on right)
Made of medium weight dark brown moleskin cloth. Lined with fine sheepskin pelts. Sleeves lined with heavy material. Has deep beaverized sheepskin collar. Woolen wind protectors in sleeves. Is fitted with belt all around and has four non-tearable, leather tipped pockets. Closes with two rows of buttons and loops which may be used from either side. Length 36 inches. Sizes 36 to 48.

No. 1885 - SHEEPLINED MOLESKIN COAT
(36 in. Heavy cloth, 4 Pockets and Belt)
(See picture on right)
Made of Heavy weight dark brown cloth. Is lined with grade A sheepskin pelts. Sleeves warmly lined with heavy cloth. Has broad beaverized sheepskin collar. Has four leather-trimmed pockets and a belt all around. Fitted with woolen wristlets in sleeves. Closes with buttons and loops in popular double breasted style. Length 36 inches. Sizes 36-48.

No. 1840 — FULL LINED 36-inch SHEEPLINED MOLESKIN COAT
(Heavy Cloth, 4 Pockets, Belt and Lining Full to Right Edge)
(See picture on left)
Made of heavy weight dark brown cloth. Is lined with selected sheepskin pelts. The sheepskin lining extends full to the right edge of coat. Fitted with deep beaverized shawl collar. Has a broad belt all around with tongueless metal buckle. Sleeves are lined with heavy cloth. The coat is equipped with 4 non-tearable leather-tipped pockets. Woolen wind protectors in sleeves. Buttoned tabs at collar. Closes with buttons and loops. Double breasted. Length 36 inches. Sizes 36 to 48.

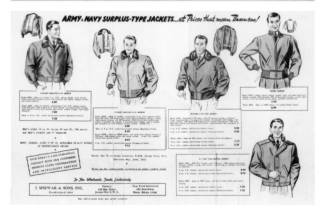

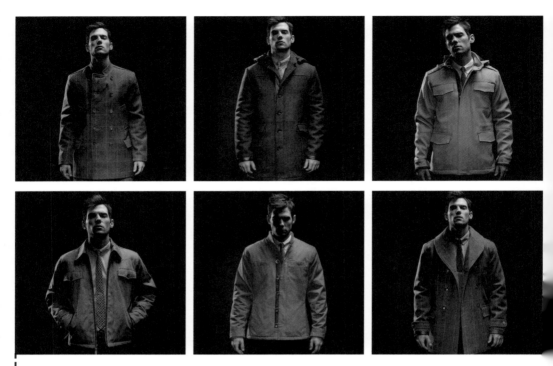

Spiewak's more classic designs, which have found fans among streetwear followers,
are largely based on items originally created for the military, including takes on the
short parka, mackinaw coat and tank jacket.

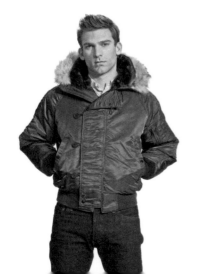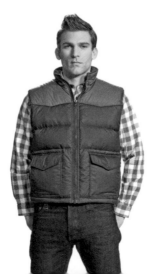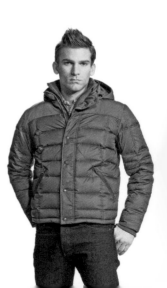

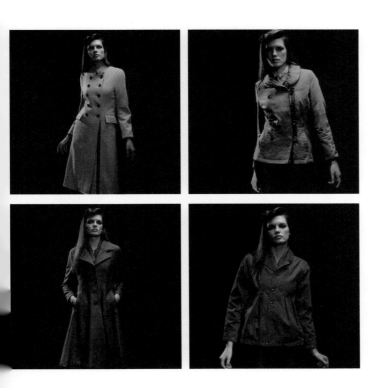

Spiewak may have outfitted the NYPD, but it has also struck up more streetwear-friendly collaborations with, among others, Kidrobot, the limited edition clothing and toymaker founded in 2002 by designer Paul Budnitz.

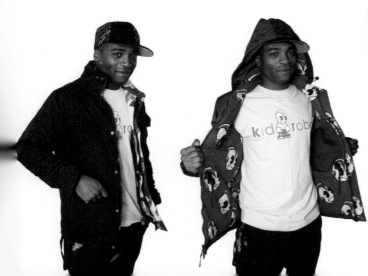

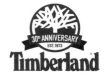

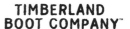

Timberland

TIMBERLAND
BOOT COMPANY™

In a market so enamoured of sneakers, for a boot to become an icon not just of the brand behind it but of streetwear at large is to pull off something of a coup. But Timberland may have achieved just this with their much-copied yellow boot. It's a statement of ruggedness, of the outdoors life (its colour is meant to mimic the shade of wheatbuck), even if it was adopted by inner-city dwellers, and widely considered a definitively American product, even if it is actually made just outside Santiago, in the Dominican Republic.

Some 80 processes and 39 components – including the leather swing-tag, which was invariably left on the boot – came together to make a chunky piece of footwear suitably proportionate to the baggy tops, sweatpants and puffa jackets with which it was often worn. A pair of 'Timbs', 'Timmies' or 'Timbos', as they were affectionately nicknamed, became especially totemic with African-American and Latino youths in New York, New Jersey and Connecticut, to the extent that, in the early to mid-1990s, stores had trouble keeping the boot in stock. Inevitably, Timberland boots achieved several laudatory nods in rap lyrics from the likes of Boot Camp Clik and the Wu-Tang Clan. "Ruff like Timberland wear, yeah/Me and the clan, and yo the Landcruisers out there," as the Clan expressed it in "Da Mystery of Chessboxin".

Although it has fought shy of being considered a streetwear brand per se, Timberland has recently taken steps at least to acknowledge its association: in 2005, with the launch of the Timberland Boot Company (a spin-off line of more upmarket and directional workwear-inspired boots, built more for style than performance); in 2006, with the acquisition of Howies, a British casualwear brand with an eco bent and connections to the BMX and snowboarding worlds; and in 2007, with the acquisition of the San Francisco skate-inspired footwear and clothing brand iPath. The same year saw perhaps the most open acceptance of its streetwear following to date: the Boroughs Project invited five artists, each representing one of New York's five boroughs, to design a limited edition Timberland boot. A further design collaboration followed, this time with New York streetwear brand Alife.

But it was the people who wore streetwear who got there before the company did, the brand inspiring hip-hop producer DeVante Swing to give young rapper Timothy Mosley the moniker 'Timbaland'. The history of Timberland, the brand, begins in

Boston, Massachusetts, in 1918, with one Nathan Swartz, who had trained as a bootmaker's stitcher, but it would be another 47 years before Timberland itself was launched. In 1952 Swartz bought half an interest in the Abington Shoe Company, and the remainder three years later, when he was joined by his son Sidney to create a family shoe business. But it took another seven years of producing for other brands before deciding to strike out with his own product.

The turning point, in 1965, was the invention of injection-moulded technology, which allowed the first fully waterproof boots to be made by fusing the soles to leather uppers without stitching. Swartz saw that this presented an opportunity to produce a boot with a claim that could set it apart from much of the competition, and in 1973, Timberlander, meaning 'man of the woods', was selected as the brand name for the lumberjack waterproof boot Swartz's company launched. The name did not catch on, but 'Timberland' did. And it was only in 1978, after phenomenal sales of the boot, that the entire business followed suit, being renamed the Timberland Company.

In 1986 Sidney took over the running of the company, introducing clothing and Timberland stores the same year and making Timberland the first boot company to advertise on US national television, a key step in transforming Timberland from a specialist, outward-bounds product to an everyday, casual one. He, in turn, was succeeded by his son Jeffrey Swartz in 1998, who launched the first Timberland licences and took the company those extra steps further, transforming it into a lifestyle brand.

The Timberland boot may have become a fashion item and part of a lifestyle brand, but its heritage is as a utility item, designed and made to be as hard-wearing as a Jeep or rucksack. Attention needs to be paid to cutting and stitching details to ensure waterproofing, for example.

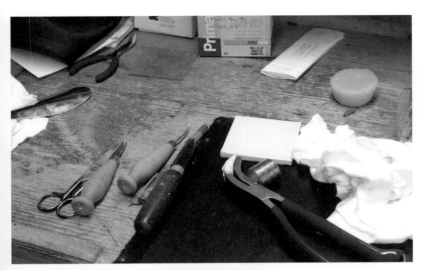

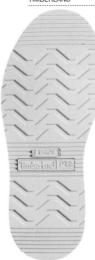

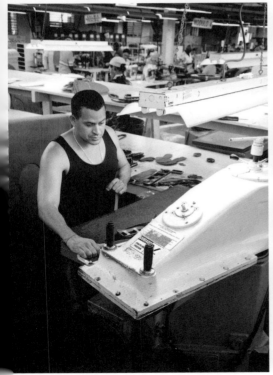

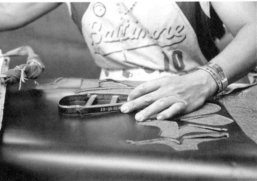

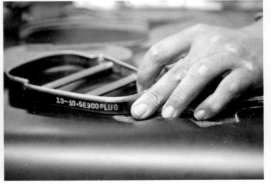

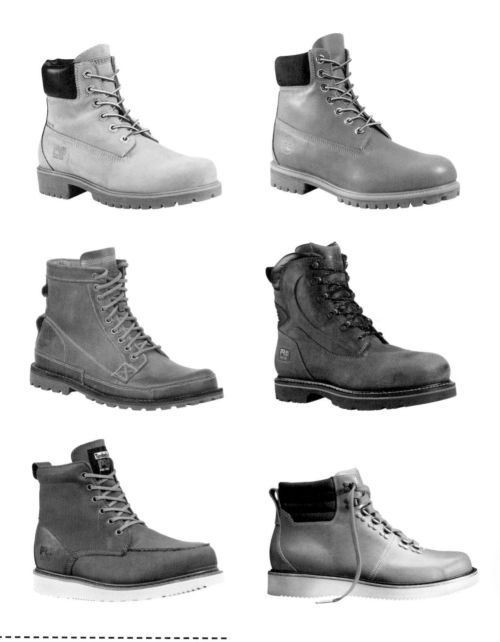

While Timberland has extended its boot repertoire to include alpine and Red Wing styles (bottom row), as well as upmarket designs from its Timberland Boot Company spin-off brand (centre row, left), its worldwide reputation has been built on one style alone: the yellow boot (main picture, opposite). It is an unlikely colour for a men's fashion icon, but icon it is.

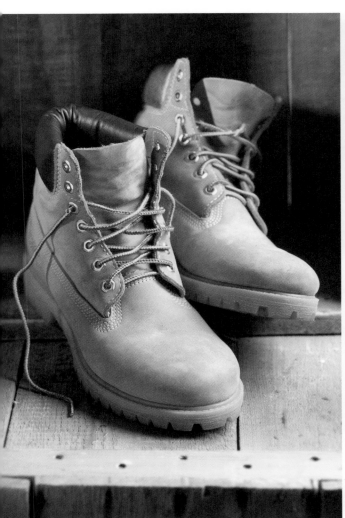

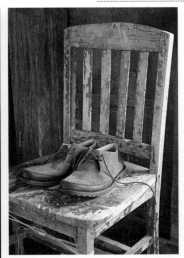

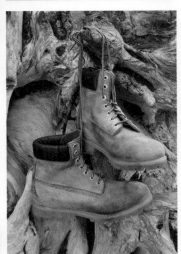

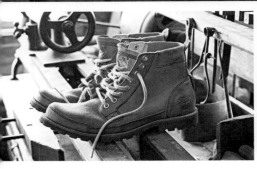

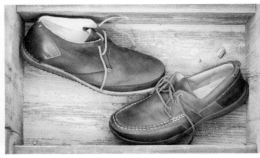

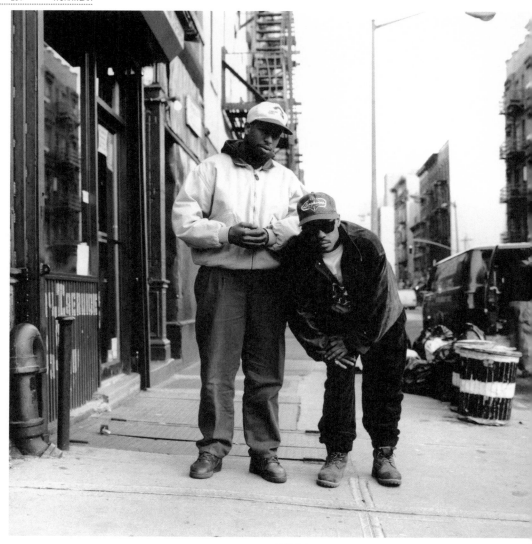

The adoption of the yellow boot by the hip-hop community – represented here by
Christopher Martin and Keith Elam of Gang Starr on a New York street in 1988
(above) and rapper and entrepreneur Jay Z (opposite, left) – has made it at home
on urban streets as in mountain backwaters. The two worlds of the great outdoors
and the urban jungle could hardly be more diverse.

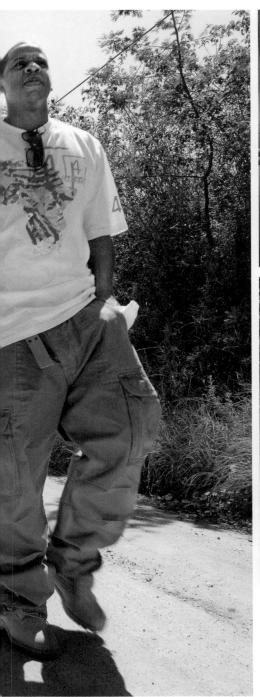

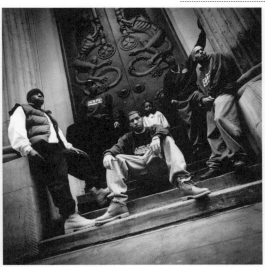

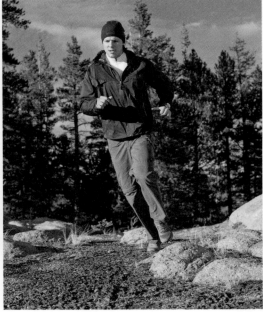

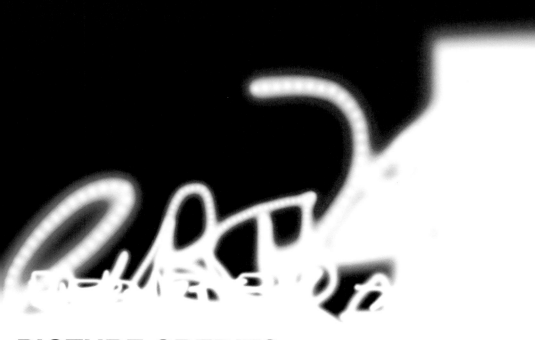

PICTURE CREDITS

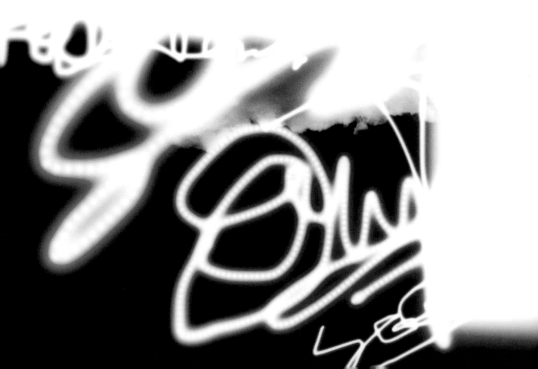

STREETWEAR

ADDICT pages 12–17
All images copyright and courtesy of Addict.

BAPE pages 9 centre, 18–21
Logo A BATHING APE®. All images ©NOWHERE CO., LTD. All rights reserved. 1993/2009.

BBC pages 22–27
Page 23 all photos Jimmy Cohrssen/www.jimmycohrssen. com; page 24, Season 7 items David Perez Shadi/www.shadinyc. com; page 24 top right, page 25 bottom, page 27 bottom P.M. Ken/www.pmken.com; page 26 Keiichi Nitta/www.keiichi-nitta.co. All product stills copyright and courtesy of Billionaire Boys Club.

EVISU pages 28–33
Page 29 second row left, third row right and bottom row, page 30 top, page 31 all images by Thomas Schlijper; page 32 top row both images by Takay, styling by Adam Howe.

FUCT pages 9 left, 34–39
Page 39, photographer Shawn Mortensen. All images copyright and courtesy of Fuct.

GOODENOUGH pages 40–45
Photographer Takashi Mizutsugi. All pictures copyright and courtesy of Tilt Corp., Ltd.

MAHARISHI pages 46–51
All images copyright and courtesy of Maharishi.

MAMBO pages 52–57
Page 53 three images above left, art by Shannon Graham; three images centre column by Wayne Golding; top right Phil Harkness. Page 54 centre right (Still Life With Franchise) Phil Harkness; page 55 all garment shots by Shannon Graham.

MECCA pages 58–63
Page 59 Rock Mecca ad campaign '01. Page 60 top row 'Trey Songz', Atlantic recording artist; page 60 bottom row 'I Rock Mecca' campaign, L–R Dave Meyers, director; Ray Cash, Ghet-O-Vision recording artist; Kwame, music producer; John Regelski, Mecca's Top Model winner. Page 61 The Saga Begins, Fall '08; models Junior and Brandon Evans. Page 62 Fall '05 collection, Rah'Saan, Renegade recording artist. Page 63 Everyday People ad campaign.

MOOKS pages 64–69
Page 66 Regeneration, concept and design by Furst Media; page 67 photography by Juan Mon.

NEIGHBORHOOD pages 70–75
Page 71 bottom row right, page 72, page 73 bottom row all, page 74 bottom row both, page 75 bottom row both by Toshiaki Shiga; page 73 top row both, page 74 top, page 75 top by Yoshiki Suzuki.

OBEY pages 8 right, 76–81
Page 77 below left by Kyle Oldoerp, all other images by Jon Furlong; page 79 top left Adam Wallacavage; centre and bottom left, centre right by Jon Furlong; bottom right by Kyle Oldoerp; page 80 by Jon Furlong.

ONE TRUE SAXON pages 82–87
All images copyright and courtesy of One True Saxon.

STUSSY pages 8 centre, 88–95
All images copyright and courtesy of Stussy.

THE HUNDREDS pages 96–101
All images copyright and courtesy of The Hundreds.

TRIPLE FIVE SOUL pages 102–107
All images copyright and courtesy of Triple Five Soul.

XLARGE pages 108–111
All images copyright and courtesy of XLarge.

ZOO YORK pages 112–117
All images copyright and courtesy of Zoo York.

SPORTSWEAR

ADIDAS pages 120–125
All images copyright and courtesy of Adidas.

BURTON pages 126–131
All images copyright and courtesy of Burton Snowboards.

CONVERSE pages 132–137
Page 133 below, page 134 images on right by David Gill.

FRED PERRY pages 138–143
Pages 140, 141 'Mods on Scooters' © Moonpix, 'Ska Girls' and 'Rude Boy Twins' © Janette Beckman. Pages 142, 143 all photography by Julian Hayr.

LACOSTE pages 144–149
All images copyright and courtesy of Lacoste.

NIKE pages 9 right, 150–155
All images copyright and courtesy of Nike.

PUMA pages 156–161
All images copyright and courtesy of Puma.

VANS pages 162–167
Pages 166 top row, 167 top left, 167 centre page by Anthony Acosta; page 166 centre left by Wynn Miller; page 166 bottom left by Ane Jens; page 167 top right by Leo Sharp.

WORKWEAR

BEN DAVIS pages 170–175
All images copyright and courtesy of Ben Davis.

CARHARTT pages 176–181
All images copyright and courtesy of Carhartt.

DICKIES pages 8 left, 182–187
All images copyright and courtesy of Dickies.

RED WING pages 188–193
All images copyright and courtesy of Red Wing.

SPIEWAK pages 194–199
Page 197 top left by Michelle LeClerc; page 198 all images, page 199 top four images by Jeffrey Westbrook; page 199 bottom two images by KidRobot.

TIMBERLAND pages 200–205
Page 204 copyright Getty Images, page 205 left copyright Corbis, page 205 top right copyright PYMCA. All other images copyright and courtesy of Timberland.

USEFUL WEBSITES

Streetwear
www.addict.co.uk
www.bape.com
www.bbcicecream.com
www.evisu.com
www.fuct.com
www.mambo.com.au
www.meccausa.com
www.mooks.com
www.neighborhood.jp
www.obeyclothing.com
www.onetruesaxon.com
www.stussy.com
www.thehundreds.com
www.triple5soul.com
www.xlarge.com
www.zooyork.com

Sportswear
www.adidas.com
www.burton.com
www.converse.com
www.fredperry.com
www.lacoste.com   www.nike.com
www.puma.com   www.vans.com

Workwear
www.bendavis.com
www.carhartt.com
www.dickies.com
www.redwingshoes.com
www.spiewak.com
www.timberland.com

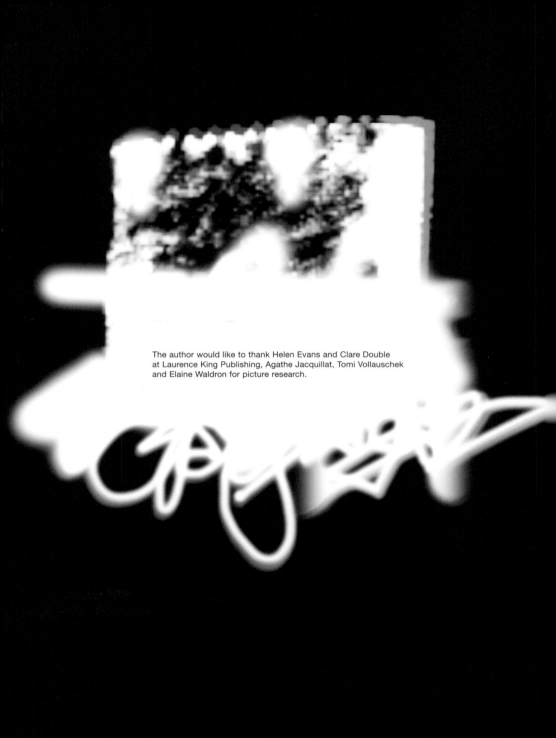

The author would like to thank Helen Evans and Clare Double
at Laurence King Publishing, Agathe Jacquillat, Tomi Vollauschek
and Elaine Waldron for picture research.